T0200672

Basic Concepts in Pharmacology

What You Need to Know for Each Drug Class

Sixth Edition

Janet L. Stringer, MD, PhD
*Visiting Associate Professor of
    Internal Medicine
University of Illinois College of
    Medicine at Urbana
Urbana, Illinois*

New York   Chicago   San Francisco   Athens   London   Madrid   Mexico City
New Delhi   Milan   Singapore   Sydney   Toronto

Basic Concepts in Pharmacology: What You Need to Know for Each Drug Class, Sixth Edition

Copyright © 2022 by McGraw Hill, LLC. All rights reserved. Printed in the United States of America. Except as permitted under the United States Copyright Act of 1976, no part of this publication may be reproduced or distributed in any form or by any means, or stored in a data base or retrieval system, without the prior written permission of the publisher.

Previous editions copyright © 2017 by McGraw-Hill Education, © 2011, 2006, 2001, 1996 by The McGraw-Hill Companies, Inc.

1 2 3 4 5 6 7 8 9   LCR   27 26 25 24 23 22

ISBN 978-1-26426484-1
MHID 1-264-26484-4

This book was set in Minion Pro by KnowledgeWorks Global Ltd.
The editors were Michael Weitz and Kim J. Davis.
The production supervisor was Catherine H. Saggese.
Project management was provided by Deepanshu Manral, KnowledgeWorks Global Ltd.

This book is printed on acid-free paper.

Library of Congress Cataloging-in-Publication Data

Names: Stringer, Janet L, author.
Title: Basic concepts in pharmacology : what you need to know for each drug
   class / Janet L Stringer.
Description: Sixth edition. | New York : McGraw Hill, [2022] | Includes
   index. | Summary: "Basic Concepts in Pharmacology: What You Need to Know
   for Each Drug Class is a review book for pharmacology designed to help
   students organize and understand the hundreds of drugs covered in
   pharmacology classes today"–Provided by publisher.
Identifiers: LCCN 2021029458 (print) | LCCN 2021029459 (ebook) | ISBN
   9781264264841 (print ; alk. paper) | ISBN 1264264844 (print; alk.
   paper) | ISBN 9781264264858 (ebook) | ISBN 1264264852 (ebook)
Subjects: MESH: Pharmacological Phenomena | Pharmaceutical Preparations
Classification: LCC RM301.14 (print) | LCC RM301.14 (ebook) | NLM QV 4 |
   DDC 615/.1–dc23
LC record available at https://lccn.loc.gov/2021029458
LC ebook record available at https://lccn.loc.gov/2021029459

McGraw Hill books are available at special quantity discounts to use as premiums and sales promotions, or for use in corporate training programs. To contact a representative, please visit the Contact Us pages at www.mhprofessional.com.

Contents

Preface   viii

1. WHERE TO START   1

PART **I**

GENERAL PRINCIPLES

2. RECEPTOR THEORY   5
   Agonists   5
   Efficacy and Potency   6
   Therapeutic Index   7
   Antagonists   7
   Inverse Agonists   9

3. ABSORPTION, DISTRIBUTION, AND CLEARANCE   10
   First-Pass Effect   10
   How Drugs Cross Membranes   10
   Bioavailability   12
   Total Body Clearance   13

4. PHARMACOKINETICS   15
   Volume of Distribution   15
   First-Order Kinetics   16
   Zero-Order Kinetics   18
   Steady-State Concentration   19
   Time Needed to Reach Steady State   20
   Loading Dose   21

5. DRUG METABOLISM AND RENAL ELIMINATION   23
   Liver Metabolism   23
   Renal Excretion   24

PART **II**

DRUGS THAT AFFECT THE AUTONOMIC NERVOUS SYSTEM

6. REVIEW OF THE AUTONOMIC NERVOUS SYSTEM   27
   Why Include This Material?   27
   Relevant Anatomy   27
   Synthesis, Storage, Release, and Removal of Transmitters   29
   Receptors   30
   General Rules of Innervation   32
   Presynaptic Receptors   33

7. CHOLINERGIC AGONISTS   35
   Organization of Class   35
   Cholinergic Agonists   36
   Cholinesterase Inhibitors   37

8. CHOLINERGIC ANTAGONISTS   40
   Organization of Class   40
   Muscarinic Antagonists   40
   Ganglionic Blockers   42
   Neuromuscular Blockers   42

9. ADRENERGIC AGONISTS   44
   Organization of Class   44
   Direct-Acting Agonists   45
   Dopamine   46
   Indirect-Acting Agents   47
   Cardiovascular Effects of Norepinephrine and Epinephrine   47

10. ADRENERGIC ANTAGONISTS   49
    Organization of Class   49
    Central Blockers   49
    α-Blockers   50
    β-Blockers   51
    Mixed α- and β-Blockers   53

PART **III**

DRUGS THAT AFFECT THE
CARDIOVASCULAR SYSTEM

11. DIURETICS   57
    Organization of Class   57
    Diuretics   57
      Inhibitors of the Na$^+$-K$^+$-2Cl$^-$ Symport
        or Loop Diuretics   58
      Inhibitors of Na$^+$/Cl$^-$ Symport or
        Thiazide Diuretics   59
      Inhibitors of Renal Epithelial Na$^+$
        Channels or K$^+$-Sparing Diuretics   60
      Mineralocorticoid Receptor Antagonists
        or Aldosterone Antagonists   60
      Inhibitors of Carbonic Anhydrase   60
      Osmotic Diuretics   61
      Inhibitor of Nonspecific Cation Channel
        or Natriuretic Peptides—Nesiritide   61

12. RAS (ACE INHIBITORS AND ARBs) AND
    CCB (CALCIUM CHANNEL BLOCKERS)   62
    Drugs That Interfere with the
      Renin-Angiotensin System   62
      Angiotensin-Converting Enzyme
        Inhibitors   62
      Angiotensin II Receptor Blockers   63
      Direct Renin Inhibitor—Aliskiren   64
    Calcium Channel Blockers   64

13. ANTIHYPERTENSIVE DRUGS   66
    Organization of Class   66
    Diuretics   67
    Drugs That Interfere with the
      Renin-Angiotensin System   67
      Inhibitors of the Renin-Angiotensin
        System   67
      Mineralocorticoid Receptor
        Antagonists (MRA)   67
      Direct Renin Inhibitor   67
    Drugs That Decrease Peripheral
      Vascular Resistance   68
      Direct Vasodilators   68
      Sympathetic Nervous System Depressants 68

14. DRUGS USED IN ISCHEMIC HEART
    DISEASE AND CONGESTIVE HEART
    FAILURE   71
    Ischemic Heart Disease   71
      Organic Nitrates   72
    Congestive Heart Failure   72
      Neurohumoral Modulation   73
      Preload Reduction   74
      Afterload Reduction   75
      Enhancement of Contractility   75
      Heart Rate Reduction   75
      SGLT2 Inhibition   76

15. ANTIARRHYTHMIC DRUGS   77
    Organization of Class   77
    Class I Drugs (Sodium Channel Blockers)   78
    Class II Drugs (β-Blockers)   79
    Class III Drugs (Potassium Channel Blockers) 80
    Class IV Drugs (Calcium Channel Blockers) 81
    Other Antiarrhythmic Drugs   81
    Drugs That Increase Heart Rate   82

16. DRUGS THAT AFFECT BLOOD   83
    Organization of Class   83
    Antiplatelet Agents   84
    Anticoagulants   85
    Thrombolytic Drugs   87
    Phosphodiesterase Inhibitors   88
    Drugs Used in the Treatment of Anemia   88
    Drugs for Sickle Cell Disease   89

17. LIPID-LOWERING DRUGS   90
    Organization of Class   90
    Additional Explanation of Mechanisms   91

PART **IV**

DRUGS THAT ACT ON THE CENTRAL
NERVOUS SYSTEM

18. DRUGS USED IN DEMENTIA   97
    Organization of Class   97
    Cholinesterase Inhibitors   97
    NMDA Blocker   98

19. ANXIOLYTIC AND HYPNOTIC DRUGS   99
    Tolerance and Dependence   99
    Organization of Class   100
    Barbiturates   101
    Benzodiazepines   102
    Buspirone   104
    Drugs for Insomnia   104
      Benzodiazepine Receptor Agonists
        (Z Compounds)   104

Melatonin Receptor Agonist   104
Orexin Receptor Antagonist   105

20. DRUGS USED IN MOOD DISORDERS   106
Organization of Antidepressants   106
Serotonin-Specific Reuptake Inhibitors   107
Serotonin/Norepinephrine Reuptake
    Inhibitors (SNRI)   108
Heterocyclics/TCAs   108
Monoamine Oxidase Inhibitors   109
Other Antidepressants   110
Drugs Used in Bipolar Disorder   111

21. DRUGS USED IN THOUGHT
    DISORDERS   112
Organization of Class   112
Typical Antipsychotics (First Generation)   113
Serotonin-Dopamine Antagonists
    (Second Generation)   114
Neuroleptic Malignant Syndrome   115

22. DRUGS FOR MOVEMENT DISORDERS   116
Therapy for Parkinson Disease   116
    Dopamine Replacement Therapy   117
    Dopamine Agonist Therapy   118
    Anticholinergic Therapy   118
Therapy for ALS and MS   119
Therapy for Duchenne Muscular
    Dystrophy and Spinal Muscular Atrophy   119

23. DRUGS FOR SEIZURE DISORDERS   121
Organization of Class   121
Important Details about the Most
    Important Drugs   122
Other Drugs to Consider   123

24. NARCOTICS (OPIATES)   125
Organization of Class   125
Actions of Morphine and
    the Other Agonists   126
Distinguishing Features of Some Agonists   127
Opioid Antagonists   128
Opioid Agonist-Antagonists   128

25. GENERAL ANESTHETICS   129
Organization of Class   129
Uptake and Distribution of
    Inhalational Anesthetics   130
Elimination of Inhalational Anesthetics   131
Potency of General Anesthetics   131
Specific Gases and Volatile Liquids   131
Specific Intravenous Agents   132

26. LOCAL ANESTHETICS   133
Organization of Class   133

Mechanism of Action   134
Special Features about Individual Agents   134

PART V
CHEMOTHERAPEUTIC AGENTS

27. INTRODUCTION TO CHEMOTHERAPY   137
Approach to the Antimicrobials   137
General Principles of Therapy   137
Definitions   138
Important Concepts to Understand   138
Classification of Antimicrobials   141

28. INHIBITORS OF CELL WALL
    SYNTHESIS   142
General Features   142
β-Lactams   142
    Penicillins   144
    Cephalosporins   145
    Carbapenems   146
    Monobactams (Aztreonam)   147
Other Inhibitors of Cell Wall Synthesis   147
    Glycopeptides   147
    Bacitracin   147
    Fosfomycin   148
    Daptomycin   148

29. PROTEIN SYNTHESIS INHIBITORS   149
General Features   149
Aminoglycosides   149
Tetracyclines   150
Macrolides   151
Streptogramins and Oxazolidinones   152
Chloramphenicol   153
Clindamycin   153

30. FOLATE ANTAGONISTS   154
Mechanism of Action   154
Selected Features   155

31. QUINOLONES AND URINARY
    TRACT ANTISEPTICS   156
Drugs in This Group   156
Quinolones   156
Methenamine   157

32. DRUGS USED IN TUBERCULOSIS
    AND LEPROSY   158
Organization of Class   158
Isoniazid   159
Rifampin   160
Pyrazinamide   160
Ethambutol   160
Dapsone   161

33. ANTIFUNGAL DRUGS 162
Organization of Class 162
Azole Antifungals 163
Polyene Antifungals 164
Echinocandins 165
Fungal Protein Inhibitors 165

34. ANTHELMINTIC DRUGS 166
Organization of Class 166
Drugs Used against Cestodes and
Trematodes 166
Drugs Used against Nematodes 167
Drugs Used against Filaria 167

35. ANTIVIRAL DRUGS 169
Organization of Class 169
Anti-HIV Drugs 170
Drugs Used in Influenza (RNA Virus) 171
Drugs Used in Hepatitis B and C 172
Other Antivirals 173

36. ANTIPROTOZOAL DRUGS 175
Organization of Class 175
Metronidazole 176
Antimalarial Agents 176
Therapeutic Considerations 177
Special Features 178

37. ANTICANCER DRUGS 179
Organization of Class 179
Terminology and General Principles
of Therapy 180
Adverse Effects 181
Cytotoxic Drugs 183
Alkylating Agents 183
Antimetabolites 184
Antibiotics and Other Natural Products 185
Other Cytotoxic Drugs 187
Hormonal Agents 187
Pathway-Targeted Therapies 188
Growth Factors and Receptors 188
Intracellular Kinases 189
Angiogenesis 189
Other Targets 190
Miscellaneous Agents 190

PART VI

DRUGS THAT AFFECT THE
ENDOCRINE SYSTEM

38. ADRENOCORTICAL HORMONES 193
Organization of Class 193

Glucocorticoids 195
Mineralocorticoids 196
Inhibitors of Adrenocorticoid Synthesis 196

39. SEX STEROIDS 197
Organization of Class 197
Estrogens 198
Antiestrogens 199
Progestins 199
Antiprogestins 200
Oral Contraceptives 200
Androgens 201
Antiandrogens 201
GnRH Agonists and Antagonists 202
PDE5 Inhibitors 202

40. THYROID AND PARATHYROID DRUGS 204
Organization of Class 204
Thyroid Replacement Therapy 205
Drugs That Are Thyroid Downers 205
Parathyroid Drugs 206

41. INSULIN, GLUCAGON, AND ORAL
HYPOGLYCEMIC DRUGS 207
Organization of Class 207
Insulins 208
Oral Hypoglycemic Agents 209
Stimulation of Insulin Release 209
Decrease Production of Glucose 210
Increase Sensitivity of Tissues to
What Insulin Is Available 210
Reduce Absorption of Glucose 211
Increase Elimination of Glucose 211

PART VII

MISCELLANEOUS DRUGS

42. HISTAMINE AND ANTIHISTAMINES 215
Organization of Class 215
H_1 Receptor Antagonists 215

43. RESPIRATORY DRUGS 217
Organization of Class 217
Bronchodilators 218
β-Agonists 218
Cholinergic Antagonists 218
Methylxanthines 218
Anti-Inflammatory Drugs 219
Inhaled Corticosteroids 219
PDE-4 Inhibitor 219
Other Approaches 219
Leukotriene Modifiers 219

Anti-IgE therapy   219
Other Biologics and Cromolyn   220
Pulmonary Hypertension   220
Cystic Fibrosis   221

44. DRUGS THAT AFFECT THE
    GI TRACT   222
    Organization of Class   222
    Drugs That Act in the Upper GI Tract   222
    Drugs That Act in the Lower GI Tract   223
      Inflammatory Bowel Disease   225

45. NONNARCOTIC ANALGESICS AND
    ANTI-INFLAMMATORY DRUGS   227
    Organization of Class   227
    Nonsteroidal Anti-Inflammatory Drugs   227
    COX-2 Inhibitors   229
    Salicylates, Including Aspirin   229
    Acetaminophen   230
    Other Drugs for Arthritis   230
    Antigout Agents   231
    Drugs Used in the Treatment of Headaches   232

46. IMMUNOSUPPRESSIVES   234
    Organization of Class   234
    Calcineurin Inhibitors   234
    Proliferation Signal Inhibitors   235
    Other Immunosupressants   235
    Biologics for Transplantation   235

47. DRUGS USED IN OSTEOPOROSIS   236
    Organization of Class   236
    Bisphosphonates   237
    Denosumab   237
    Parathyroid Hormone   237
    Selective Estrogen Receptor Modulators   237
    Calcitonin   238
    Sclerostin Inhibitor   238

48. TOXICOLOGY AND POISONING   239
    Principles of Toxicology   239
    General Principles in the Treatment
      of Poisoning   239
    Specific Antidotes   240

Index   242

Preface

Basic Concepts in Pharmacology: What You Need to Know for Each Drug Class is not a conventional review book for pharmacology. It is a book to help you organize your attack on the hundreds of drugs covered in pharmacology classes today. Our survey for the first edition of this book made it clear that it is the number of drugs in a particular class that students find overwhelming. This fear causes many students to lose focus on the most important part of pharmacology—the concepts.

Because this is not a review book, I will not be covering each and every drug currently available. Instead, I will try to provide a way to organize and condense the amount of material that needs to be memorized. In addition, certain concepts and definitions will be explained. Along the way we will need to review some biochemistry and physiology, reinforcing previously learned concepts.

This book is organized so that the reader can focus on the highlights and decide whether or not to read the more detailed description. Information in the boxes is key. If you know the information in the box, skip to the next one. If you don't know the information, read the text that follows it. This book is intended to help you organize your study and avoid any extra hours spent on less important trivia, so you should approach the book in the same way.

Some drug names appear in capital letters. Although somewhat of an arbitrary choice, these drug names seem to be the most important to know. If you have time and energy to learn only three names in a particular drug class, learn the ones that appear in capital letters. Because students are expected to know only generic names of drugs, only generic names are used throughout this text.

Where to Start

Although many pharmacology students are able to memorize an incredible amount of information, there is a limit to what even the best students can learn. Therefore, you must try to organize the material in a way that minimizes the amount of information you have to memorize. Usually this means grouping drugs and making associations.

> The best approach is to learn drugs by their class.

New drugs will be introduced during your lifetime and even during your training, so it is necessary to develop a flexible framework for drug information.

From a student's perspective, it is often very difficult to know what is a priority and what can be skipped. Textbooks are usually not helpful in guiding students because of the way they are organized. They give general information about the pathophysiology or the drug class, followed by details about each individual agent in the class. This is an efficient way to be thorough, and it is very useful when you need to go back and look up a detail about a drug. It is not, however, as useful for the beginning student who must start from scratch.

To help you decide what is the most important information, I have developed a trivia sorter.

Trivia Sorter: Generic

1. The mechanism of action for the <u>class</u> of drug.

2. Properties or effects those are common to <u>all</u> drugs in the class.

3. Is (are) the drug(s) the *drug of choice* for some disorder or symptom?

4. Name recognition—what drugs are in this class?

5. Unique features about single drugs in the class.

6. Are there any side effects (rare or not) that may be *fatal*?

7. Drug interactions.

8. Rare side effects or actions that are common to all drugs in the class.

9. Rare side effects or actions for single drugs in the class.

10. Other facts such as: percentage of drug that is metabolized versus excretion unchanged, half-life of each drug, teratogenicity of each drug, structural features of individual drugs.

This generic trivia sorter will not work for all drug classes. Therefore, for each class I will indicate the way I have organized the attack on the drugs in that group. For example, the mechanism of action of the antiepileptic drugs is not clear, so you will have to skip step 1 and go to step 2. The antiarrhythmic agents are classified and grouped according to their mechanism of action, so that should be the number 1 item you learn.

You can also determine your own trivia level. I would suggest at least through number 6. If you have the time and inclination to learn more details, you will need to consult your favorite textbook.

Because the *drug of choice* is often very important to know, these drugs are included in the boxes that appear throughout the book. However, these are subject to change, so you should confirm that the drug is still the drug of choice during class or from your textbook. Fatal side effects, even if rare, are important to know for your patients' safety. I will try to point out some, but others may come up in class or in your textbook. If so, make a note to learn them.

Name recognition is a slightly different matter. From my own experience as well as that of many medical students, when an unfamiliar drug name appears in an exam, panic sets in and the question is usually skipped or answered incorrectly. However, if the drug class is known, often the question becomes simple. I recommend to students, who are having trouble with drug name recognition, to make flash cards (or lists) with only the drug name on one side and the drug class on the other side. Skip the easy ones. Quiz yourself during breakfast or during breaks between classes. As you learn the drugs, take them off your list or remove the card from the stack. Occasionally put these names back and review all together. If you only get a few more questions right on an examination or on the boards or have to look up one less drug after rounds, the few minutes that this takes will have been worth it.

The issue of drug names has become much more interesting and difficult in recent years. In the past (with some exceptions), most of the drugs with the same mechanism had the same ending to their names. Examples, the "-cillin" group is all penicillins (antibiotics) and the "-olol" group is all the β-blockers. Now we have all the "-mab" drugs, which are <u>m</u>onoclonal <u>a</u>nti<u>b</u>odies, and the "-ib" drugs (most commonly -nib), which are (mostly) kinase inhibitors and sometimes called small molecule inhibitors. These drugs are used for treatment of cancer, respiratory disease, GI diseases, immune system diseases, etc. Thus, the ending of the drug name no longer indicates, or even hints at, what it might be used for. In addition, for the monoclonal antibodies, the two letters preceding the "mab" are used to indicate whether the antibody is fully humanized (-mumab), has the antigen-binding region from a mouse antibody (-zumab), is a chimeric with human and mouse parts (-ximab), or is entirely mouse (-omab). The two letters before these are supposed to indicate the organ system that is the target for the antibody. This results in long names that are of little help for the student, except that you should be able to identify that the drug is a monoclonal antibody or kinase inhibitor.

The names for the monoclonal antibodies often are presented with a four-letter extension (e.g., caplacizumab-yhdp). This four-letter suffix has no pronunciation or meaning. The suffix has been added to distinguish reference products from biosimilar products.

PART I General Principles

CHAPTER 2:   Receptor Theory   05

CHAPTER 3:   Absorption, Distribution, and Clearance   10

CHAPTER 4:   Pharmacokinetics   15

CHAPTER 5:   Drug Metabolism and Renal Elimination   23

Receptor Theory

> Agonists
> Efficacy and Potency
> Therapeutic Index
> Antagonists
> Inverse Agonists

AGONISTS

> An agonist is a compound that binds to a receptor and produces the biological response.

A drug receptor is a specialized target macromolecule that binds a drug and mediates its pharmacological action. These receptors may be enzymes, nucleic acids, or specialized membrane-bound proteins. The formation of the drug-receptor complex leads to a biological response. The magnitude of the response is proportional to the number of drug-receptor complexes. A common way to present the relationship between the drug concentration and the biological response is with a concentration- (or dose-) response curve (Figure 2–1). In many textbooks, you will see both dose-response curves and concentration-response curves. Because the biological effect is more closely related to the plasma concentration than to the dose, I will show concentration-response curves in this chapter.

An agonist can be a drug or the endogenous ligand for the receptor. Increasing concentrations of the agonist will increase the biological response until there are no more receptors for the agonist to bind or a maximal response has been reached.

> A partial agonist produces the biological response but cannot produce 100% of the biological response even at very high doses.

Figure 2–1 shows concentration response curves and compares a partial agonist with a "full" agonist.

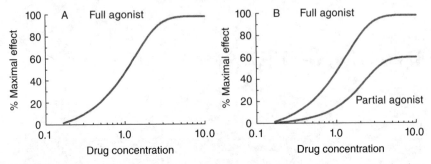

FIGURE 2–1 In A, the concentration-response curve for a full agonist is presented. The drug can produce a maximal effect. In B, the concentration-response curve for a partial agonist is also shown. In this case, the partial agonist is able to produce only 60% of the maximal response.

EFFICACY AND POTENCY

Efficacy and *potency* are terms used for comparisons between drugs.

> *Efficacy* is the maximal response a drug can produce. *Potency* is a measure of the dose that is required to produce a response.

For example, one drug (drug A) produces complete eradication of premature ventricular contractions (PVCs) at a dose of 10 mg. A second drug (drug B) produces complete eradication of PVCs at a dose of 20 mg. Therefore, both drugs have the same efficacy (complete eradication of PVCs), but drug A is more potent than drug B. It takes less of drug A to produce the same effect. A third drug (drug C) can reduce the PVCs by only 60%, and it takes a dose of 50 mg to achieve that effect. Therefore, drug C has less efficacy and less potency in the reduction of PVCs compared with both drugs A and B.

Potency and efficacy are usually shown graphically (Figure 2–2).

> Potency is often expressed as the dose of a drug required to achieve 50% of the desired therapeutic effect. This is denoted by ED_{50} (effective dose).

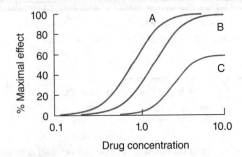

FIGURE 2–2 Concentration-response curves for drugs A, B, and C are presented. Drugs A and B have equal efficacy, but drug A is more potent than drug B. Drug C is less efficacious and less potent than either drug A or drug B.

THERAPEUTIC INDEX

> Therapeutic index is a measure of drug safety. A drug with a higher therapeutic index is safer than one with a lower therapeutic index.

That statement is true no matter what textbook you consult. However, the definition of therapeutic index may vary depending on the book. Usually,

$$\text{Therapeutic index} = \frac{LD_{50}}{ED_{50}}$$

The LD_{50} is the dose that kills 50% of the animals that receive it. Sometimes the TD_{50} is used in place of the LD_{50}. The TD_{50} is the dose that is toxic in 50% of the animals that receive it. Death is the ultimate toxicity.

The therapeutic index is sometimes confused with the therapeutic window. The therapeutic window is the range of plasma concentrations of a drug that will elicit the desired response in a population of patients.

ANTAGONISTS

> Antagonists block or reverse the effect of agonists. They have no effect of their own.

Binding of an antagonist to a receptor does not produce a biological effect. The antagonist can block the effect of an agonist, or it can reverse the effect of an agonist. An example of an antagonist is naloxone, an opioid antagonist (see Chapter 24). Naloxone has no effect of its own but will completely reverse the effects of any opioid agonist that has been administered. Sometimes the antagonist reverses or blocks the effect of endogenously produced compounds, such as epinephrine or norepinephrine. This is the mechanism of action of β-blockers.

> Competitive antagonists make the agonist look less potent by shifting the dose-response curve to the right.

Because antagonists have no effect of their own, we need to consider their effect on the agonist. In the graph in Figure 2–3, we determined the biological effect produced by increasing concentrations of agonist. We then repeated the same experiment in the presence of a fixed concentration of an antagonist. This shifted the curve to the right, making the agonist look less potent.

This is easy to remember and understand. These antagonists are competitive; that is, they compete for the same site on the receptor that the agonist wants. If the agonist wins, a response is produced. If the antagonist wins, no response is produced. As we increase the concentration of agonist, we increase the odds that an

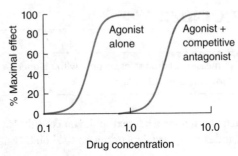

FIGURE 2–3 In this graph the concentration-response curve for an agonist alone is presented. When the effect of the agonist is tested in the presence of a fixed concentration of a competitive antagonist, the agonist appears less potent. The same maximal effect is achieved, but it takes higher doses to do so.

agonist molecule will win the receptor spot and produce an effect. At a high enough agonist concentration, the poor antagonist doesn't have a chance at the receptor; it is simply outnumbered.

> A noncompetitive antagonist reduces the maximal response that an agonist can produce.

Let's repeat the earlier experiment. We first determine the biological effect produced by increasing concentrations of an agonist. We repeat these measurements in the presence of a fixed concentration of a noncompetitive antagonist (Figure 2–4). Increasing concentrations of the agonist cannot overcome this blockade. Therefore, the maximal biological response produced by the agonist appears to have decreased because of our addition of the noncompetitive antagonist.

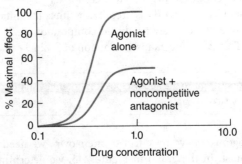

FIGURE 2–4 The concentration-response curve for the same agonist alone is presented. Then the activity of the agonist is tested in the presence of a fixed concentration of noncompetitive antagonist. In this instance the maximal response is reduced.

There are a number of molecular mechanisms by which noncompetitive antagonists can reduce the maximal effect. They can irreversibly bind to the receptor so that the agonist cannot be competed off. They can bind to a site different from the agonist and prevent either agonist binding or the agonist effect. Some books will use different terminology, such as uncompetitive, for the different mechanisms.

INVERSE AGONISTS

> Inverse (or reverse) agonists have opposite effects from those of full agonists. They are not the same as antagonists, which block the effects of both agonists and inverse agonists.

Originally, the term *inverse agonist* was used to describe the action of some drugs on conductance through ligand-gated ion channels. Most ion channels have a basal rate of opening and closing. Agonists will increase the relative amount of time the channel is in the open state compared to the basal rate. Inverse agonists will decrease the amount of time the channel is open compared to the basal rate. At the $GABA_A$ receptor-channel complex, agonists increase the amount of chloride that moves into the neuron and will hyperpolarize it. Overall, this leads to sedation. An inverse agonist will decrease the amount of chloride that moves into the neuron, which will result in a depolarization compared to the resting state. Overall, this leads to an increase in excitability and can cause seizures.

Some G protein–coupled receptors have basal activity in that they are in an equilibrium between an active and inactive states. Inverse agonists bind to the receptor and tip the equilibrium toward the inactive state, while agonists bind the receptor and tip the equilibrium toward the active state. For there to be an inverse agonist in a receptor system, there must be activity in the basal, resting state in the absence of any ligand.

While the net physiologic result of giving an inverse agonist and an antagonist may be the same, the molecular mechanism is not. Antagonists bind to the receptor, but they have no effect on the basal state. They do, however, block the effects of both agonists and inverse agonists (Figure 2–5).

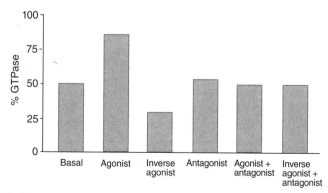

FIGURE 2–5 This graph illustrates the concept of an inverse agonist. Basal GTPase activity is compared with activity in the presence of an agonist and an inverse agonist. An antagonist has no effect on GTPase activity and completely blocks the effects of both the agonist and inverse agonist.

3

Absorption, Distribution, and Clearance

First-Pass Effect
How Drugs Cross Membranes
Bioavailability
Total Body Clearance

FIRST-PASS EFFECT

> The liver is a metabolic machine and often inactivates drugs on their way from the gastrointestinal (GI) tract to the body. This is called the *first-pass effect*.

Orally administered drugs are absorbed from the gastrointestinal (GI) tract. The blood from the GI tract then travels through the liver, the great chemical plant in the body. Many drugs that undergo liver metabolism will be extensively metabolized during this passage from the GI tract to the body. This effect of liver metabolism is called the *first-pass effect*.

HOW DRUGS CROSS MEMBRANES

There are several useful routes of drug administration, but almost all require that the drug cross a biological membrane to reach its site of action.

> Drugs cross membranes by passive diffusion or active transport.

This statement is somewhat simplified, but it provides a useful starting point. Passive diffusion requires a concentration gradient across the membrane. The vast majority of drugs gain access to their site of action by this method.

> A drug tends to pass through membranes if it is uncharged.

Uncharged drugs are more lipid soluble than charged drugs. In addition, most drugs are weak acids or weak bases.

For a weak acid, when the pH is less than the pK, the protonated form (nonionized) predominates. When the pH is greater than the pK, the unprotonated (ionized) form predominates.

$$HA \leftrightarrows H^+ + A^-$$

Weak acids are hydrogen ion donors; they are happy to give up a hydrogen ion and become charged. If you have trouble remembering whether they become charged or uncharged after donating their hydrogen ion, think of a strong acid, such as HCl. As you know, when you put HCl into water, it immediately turns into H^+ and Cl^-. Use this example to remember that weak acids donate a hydrogen ion and become charged.

Remember the pK? That is the equilibrium constant (of course, the p means we've taken the negative log of the equilibrium constant). When the pH is equal to the pK, there are equal amounts of weak acid in the ionized and nonionized forms. If we decrease the pH by adding more H^+, we will drive the equilibrium for the weak acid more to the left, which is the nonionized (uncharged) form.

If we take away H^+, making the pH higher, we will drive the equilibrium toward the right. This increases the concentration of the ionized form of the weak acid (Figure 3–1).

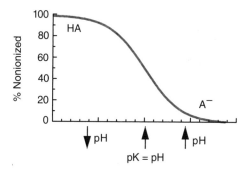

FIGURE 3-1 The relationship between the pH and the degree of ionization of a weak acid is presented. When the pH is higher than the pK for the acid, the charged form of the acid predominates.

For a weak base, when the pH is less than the pK, the ionized form (protonated) predominates. When the pH is greater than the pK, the unprotonated (nonionized) form predominates.

Weak bases are the opposite of weak acids. A weak base is a hydrogen ion acceptor. If a loose hydrogen ion seeks to join it, the base may accept it. If it accepts the hydrogen ion, it becomes charged.

$$B + H^+ \leftrightarrows BH^+$$

Adding H^+ to lower the pH will drive the equilibrium to the right toward the protonated (charged) form. Removing H^+ to raise the pH will drive the equilibrium to the left toward the uncharged form (unprotonated) of the base (Figure 3–2).

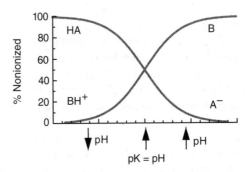

FIGURE 3–2 In this graph the effects of pH on the degree of ionization of both a weak acid and a weak base are presented.

To test your understanding of this, try out these questions. Answers appear at the bottom of the page.*

1. In the intestine (pH 8.0), which will be better absorbed, a weak acid (pK 6.8) or a weak base (pK 7.1)?

2. If we alkalinize the urine to a pH of 7.8, will a lower or higher percentage of a weak acid (pK 7.1) be ionized, compared with when the urine pH was 7.2?

BIOAVAILABILITY

> *Bioavailability* is the amount of drug that is absorbed after administration by route X compared with the amount of drug that is absorbed after intravenous (IV) administration. X is any route of drug administration other than IV.

Example: Suppose you are testing a compound in clinical trials. You have tentatively named this compound "Newdrug." Newdrug is administered orally and plasma levels determine that only 75% of the oral dose reaches the circulation. Compared with intravenous (IV) administration where 100% of the dose reaches the circulation, the bioavailability of Newdrug is 0.75 or 75%. In the case of

*Answers: (1) a weak base; (2) higher, because more weak acid will be ionized the more the pH exceeds the pK.

hypothetical Newdrug, you discover that some of the drug is inactivated by the acid in the stomach. You redesign the pill with a coating that is stable in acid but dissolves in the more basic pH of the small intestine. The bioavailability of the drug increases to 95%. Newdrug becomes a best-selling product (Figure 3–3).

$$\text{Bioavailability} = \frac{AUC_{oral}}{AUC_{IV}}$$

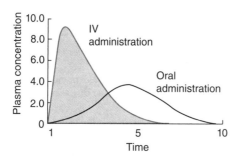

FIGURE 3–3 The plasma concentration plotted against the time and the area under the curve (AUC) is an indication of bioavailability. In this graph, an orally administered drug is compared with the same drug administered intravenously.

TOTAL BODY CLEARANCE

Clearance is a term that indicates the rate at which a drug is cleared from the body. It is defined as the volume of plasma from which all drug is removed in a given time. Thus, the units for clearance are given in volume per unit time.

Clearance is an odd term, mostly because of the units used to report it. It is not intuitive. Try the following exercise as a way to remember the units.

Suppose we have a 10-L aquarium that contains 10,000 mg of crud. The concentration is 1 mg/mL. Clearance is 1 L/h. In other words, the aquarium filter and pump clear 1 L of water in an hour. At the end of the first hour, 1000 mg of crud has been removed from the aquarium (1000 mL of 1 mg/mL). The aquarium thus has 9000 mg of crud remaining, for a concentration of 0.9 mg/mL. At the end of the second hour, 900 mg of crud has been removed (1000 mL of 0.9 mg/mL). The aquarium now has 8100 mg of crud remaining, for a concentration of 0.81 mg/mL. This process continues forever. Notice that the time to clear this particular aquarium is not 10 hours. It would take 10 hours (10 L at 1 L/h) if the clean water was pumped into another container. In the case of clearance in the aquarium, however, the clean water is returned to the tank and dilutes the remaining crud (Figure 3–4). The same principle holds true for clearance of a drug from the human body.

Pump filter rate = clearance

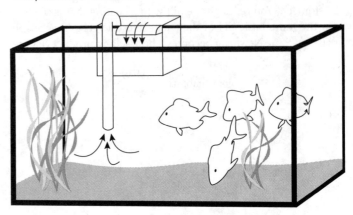

FIGURE 3–4 Clearance is very much like an aquarium pump. The pump cleans a fixed amount of water in the aquarium in a set amount of time (the clearance). The clean water returns to the aquarium, diluting the remaining water.

A more official definition is the following equation:

$$\text{Clearance} = \frac{\text{Rate of removal of drug (mg/min)}}{\text{Plasma concentration of drug (mg/mL)}}$$

Notice that this equation gives you units of milliliters per minute (mL/min) or volume per unit time.

Total body clearance is the sum of the clearances from the various organs involved in drug metabolism and elimination.

Pharmacokinetics

- Volume of Distribution
- First-Order Kinetics
- Zero-Order Kinetics
- Steady-State Concentration
- Time Needed to Reach Steady State
- Loading Dose

Pharmacokinetics is the mathematical description of the rate and extent of uptake, distribution, and elimination of drugs in the body.

VOLUME OF DISTRIBUTION

Volume of distribution (V_D) is a calculation of the apparent volume in which a drug is dissolved.

This definition assumes that the drug is evenly distributed and that metabolism or elimination has not taken place. In reality, it does not correspond to any real volume:

$$\text{Volume of distribution } (V_D) = \frac{\text{Dose (mg)}}{\text{Plasma concentration (mg/mL)}}$$

This equation is very easy to remember. Suppose you take 1000 mg of sugar and dissolve it into a beaker of water. After it has dissolved, you take a sample of water (let's say, 10 mL) and determine the concentration of sugar in that sample (e.g., 1 mg/mL). From this finding you can calculate the volume of water in which the sugar was dissolved, as follows:

$$1 \text{ mg/mL} = 1000 \text{ mg/volume of water}$$

Thus,

$$\text{Volume} = \frac{1000 \text{ mg}}{1 \text{ mg/mL}} = 1000 \text{ mL}$$

In this case the volume was 1000 mL or 1 L. If you keep the units straight, the equation does not need to be memorized.

Try another one. Suppose 500 mg of "Newdrug" is administered to a medical student. The plasma concentration is 0.01 mg/mL. What is the volume of distribution?*

The volume of distribution is rather large. Your selected medical student is not, however, a huge water balloon. The only explanation is that the drug is hiding at some place in the body where it is not recorded by the measurement of plasma concentration. The drug could be lipid soluble and stored in fat, or it could be bound to plasma proteins. As this example shows, the volume of distribution is a hypothetical volume and not a real volume.

The volume of distribution gives a rough accounting of where a drug goes in the body, especially if you have a feel for the various body fluid compartments and their sizes (Figure 4–1). In addition, it can be used to calculate the dose of a drug needed to achieve a desired plasma concentration.

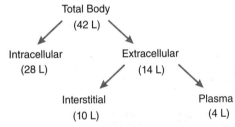

FIGURE 4–1 The various body fluid compartments for a standard 70-kg man are illustrated in this figure.

FIRST-ORDER KINETICS

The order of a reaction refers to the way in which the concentration of drug or reactant influences the rate of a chemical reaction. For most drugs, we need only consider first-order and zero-order.

> Most drugs disappear from plasma by processes that are concentration-dependent, which results in first-order kinetics. With first-order elimination, a constant percentage of the drug is lost per unit time. An elimination rate constant can be described.

The elimination rate constant is k_e (units are 1/time). On a log plot, the curve is linear and the slope of the line is equal to $k_e/2.303$. (The factor 2.303 converts from natural log to base 10 log units.)

---

*Answer: 50,000 mL or 50 L.

The half-life ($t_{1/2}$) is the period of time required for the concentration of a drug to decrease by one-half.

The half-life, or $t_{1/2}$, is shown graphically in Figure 4–2.

The half-life is constant and related to k_e for drugs that have first-order kinetics.
$$t_{1/2} = 0.693/k_e$$

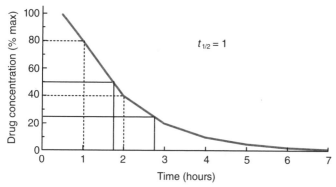

FIGURE 4–2 The determination of the half-life ($t_{1/2}$) of a drug with first-order kinetics is illustrated. The drug concentration is graphed against the time. The time it takes for the concentration to decrease by 50% is indicated at two places on the curve. The $t_{1/2}$ is the same for both determinations.

First-order elimination rate
= Rate constant × Plasma concentration × Volume of distribution
= k(1/min) × C_p(mg/mL) × V_D(mL)
= mg/min

Clearance of a drug is different from the elimination rate.

Remember clearance? As explained in Chapter 3, it's the volume of fluid cleared of a drug per unit time. In contrast, the elimination rate is the rate of removal of drug with the units of weight per unit time. For drugs with first-order kinetics, clearance and elimination rate are related, as shown in the following equation:

$$\text{Clearance} = \frac{\text{Rate of removal of drug (mg/min)}}{\text{Plasma concentration of drug (mg/mL)}}$$

For drugs with first-order kinetics, the V_D, $t_{1/2}$, k_e, and clearance are all interrelated.

ZERO-ORDER KINETICS

> Drugs that saturate routes of elimination disappear from plasma in a non–concentration-dependent manner, which is zero-order kinetics.

Metabolism in the liver, which involves specific enzymes, is one of the most important factors that contribute to a drug having zero-order kinetics. The most common examples of drugs that have zero-order kinetics are aspirin, phenytoin, and ethanol. Many drugs will show zero-order kinetics at high, or toxic, concentrations.

> For drugs with zero-order kinetics, a constant amount of drug is lost per unit time. The half-life is not constant but depends on the concentration.

The higher the concentration, the longer the $t_{1/2}$. This is illustrated in Figure 4–3. Because the $t_{1/2}$ changes as the drug concentration declines, the zero-order $t_{1/2}$ has little practical significance.

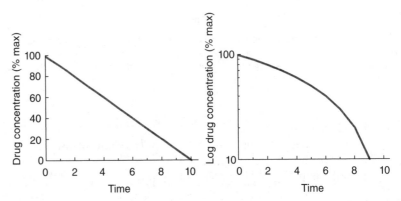

FIGURE 4–3 A drug showing zero-order elimination kinetics is illustrated here. On the left, the drug concentration is plotted on a linear scale and on the right, on a logarithmic scale. Notice that drugs with zero-order kinetics show a straight line on the linear scale. Try calculating the half-life of this drug in at least two different places. Do you get the same value?

> Zero-order kinetics is also known as nonlinear or dose-dependent kinetics.

You will see the terms *zero-order*, *nonlinear*, and *dose-dependent* used interchangeably in the medical literature. The term *dose-dependent* refers to drugs that are first-order at lower doses and switch to zero-order at higher doses (often in the therapeutic range). Therefore, the kinetics of these drugs are dose-dependent.

Nonlinear refers to the fact that drugs with zero-order kinetics do not show a linear relationship between drug dose and plasma concentration.

STEADY-STATE CONCENTRATION

> With multiple dosing, or a continuous infusion, a drug will accumulate until the amount administrated per unit time is equal to the amount eliminated per unit time. The plasma concentration at this point is called the *steady-state concentration* (C_{ss}).

Rarely are drugs given as a single dose. Normally repeated doses are given, and sometimes drugs are given as a continuous intravenous (IV) infusion. When a drug is given as a continuous infusion, it will increase in concentration in the blood until the rate of elimination is equal to the infusion rate (Figure 4–4).

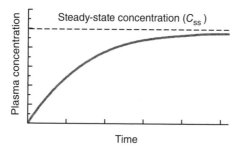

FIGURE 4–4 A continuous intravenous (IV) infusion of a drug was started at the beginning point of the graph. The concentration of the drug in the plasma was followed over time. When the amount delivered in a unit of time is equal to the amount eliminated in the same time unit, the plasma concentration is said to have reached steady state.

Let's consider a patient who has no drug in his system. You start an IV infusion at 100 mg/min. At first the plasma level will be low and the infusion rate will be greater than the elimination rate. The plasma level will rise relatively quickly. Remember that the elimination rate is proportional to the plasma concentration of the drug, so as the concentration rises so does the elimination rate. As the elimination rate increases with the increasing plasma concentration, the rate of increase in the plasma level will slow down. At steady state, the infusion rate and the elimination rate are equal.

For an IV infusion,

$$C_{SS} = \frac{\text{Infusion rate (mg/min)}}{\text{Clearance (mL/min)}} = \text{mg/mL}$$

Notice the direct relationship between C_{ss} and the infusion rate (assuming clearance is constant). If we double the infusion rate, the C_{ss} doubles.

There is also a concentration at steady state for repeated doses. Some textbooks call this an average concentration (C_{av}). With multiple dosing schedules, we normally assume that early doses of the drug do not affect the pharmacokinetics of subsequent doses. Generally, we also give equal doses at equal time intervals.

> Repeated dosing is associated with peak and trough plasma concentrations.

With repeated dosing, the concentration fluctuates around a mean (steady-state value) with peak and trough values. Here, steady state is achieved when the dose administered and the amount eliminated in a given dosing interval is the same (Figure 4–5). The goal is to have the concentration remain within the therapeutic window, where it is effective, but not toxic. Sometimes this is not the case with a chosen dosing schedule. Either the peak reaches into the toxic range, in which case the patient experiences side effects, or the trough drops too low and the drug is no longer effective. Both of these problems can be solved by adjusting the dose and dosing schedule.

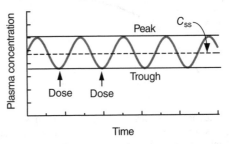

FIGURE 4–5 This graph shows the change in concentration with repeated doses. Peak and trough levels are indicated, as well as the steady-state concentration (or average concentration).

TIME NEEDED TO REACH STEADY STATE

So far we've focused on the concentration at steady state. Now let's consider the time it takes to reach this steady-state concentration.

> The time needed to reach steady state depends only on the half-life of the drug. Ninety percent of steady state is reached in 3.3 half-lives.

There is a good bit of math behind these numbers, which you can read about elsewhere if you want. Remember that to have a half-life, the drug has to follow first-order elimination kinetics.

The bottom line is that during each half-life, 50% of the change from the starting point to C_{ss} is achieved. After one half-life, we gain 50% of the C_{ss}. We have 50%

of the distance remaining. In the next half-life, we will gain 50% of this remaining distance, or 1/2 of 50%, which is 25%. So, after two half-lives, we will be 75% of the way to steady state. If you repeat this several times, you can generate Table 4–1. Notice that after five half-lives, we are still approaching steady state.

TABLE 4–1 Percentage of Steady State (C_{ss}) Achieved after Every Half-Life ($t_{1/2}$)

No. of $t_{1/2}$	% C_{ss}
1	50
2	75
3	88
3.3	90
4	94
5	97

When asked the question, how long does it take to get to steady state, some sources accept 3.3 half-lives (90% of C_{ss}), whereas others use 4 half-lives (94% of C_{ss}), and still others accept 5 half-lives (97% of C_{ss}). Check your textbook or lecture notes.

LOADING DOSE

If the half-life of a drug is relatively long, such as ~6 days for digitoxin, it will take quite a long time for the drug concentration to reach steady state (about four times the half-life). For digitoxin, this would take over 3 weeks. Sometimes the patient can't wait that long for the therapeutic effect to occur. In these instances, a loading dose is used.

A loading dose is a single large dose of a drug that is used to raise the plasma concentration to a therapeutic level more quickly than would occur through repeated smaller doses.

A single dose of a drug can be given that will result in the desired plasma concentration. This dose is called a loading dose if followed by repeated doses or a continuous infusion that will maintain the plasma concentration at the desired level (termed maintenance doses).

As you can see in Figure 4–6, as the concentration begins to decline after the loading dose, the concentration contributed by the continuous infusion begins to increase.

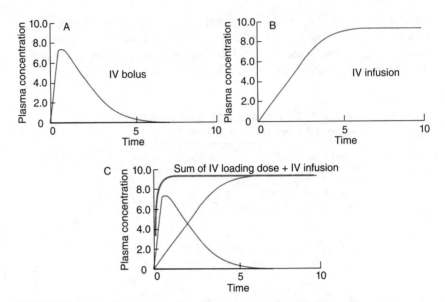

FIGURE 4–6 In A, the change in drug concentration as a function of time after an intravenous (IV) bolus is presented. In B, the change in drug concentration as a function of time after the start of a continuous IV infusion is presented. In C, both the bolus and the continuous infusion are given at time 0. The IV bolus is the loading dose. Notice how quickly the plasma concentration reaches the steady-state concentration with this technique.

Drug Metabolism and Renal Elimination

Liver Metabolism
Renal Excretion

LIVER METABOLISM

The liver is a major site for drug metabolism. The goal of metabolism is to produce metabolites that are polar or charged and can be eliminated by the kidney. Lipid-soluble agents are metabolized by the liver using two general sets of reactions, called *phase I* and *phase II*.

> Phase I reactions frequently involve the P-450 system. Phase II reactions are conjugations, mostly with glucuronide.

Phase I reactions convert lipophilic molecules into more polar molecules by introducing or unmasking a polar functional group, such as an —OH or —NH_2. Most of these reactions utilize the microsomal P-450 enzymes.

Phase I reactions are the basis of a number of drug interactions. There are a whole series of cytochrome P-450 enzymes that can be inhibited or induced. Of these, CYP3A4 plays a role in the metabolism of about 50% of the drugs that are currently prescribed. Inhibition or induction of CYP3A4 by one drug will affect the levels of any other drug that is also metabolized by CYP3A4. For example, rifampin induces CYP3A4 that can increase metabolism of estrogen, thus reducing the effectiveness of birth control pills. Some textbooks include lists of drugs that inhibit or induce CYP3A4. Don't try to memorize these lists. Be aware of the potential problem and learn the most commonly interacting drugs as you gain experience. There are also known genetic variations in levels of CYP450 enzymes.

Phase II reactions are conjugation reactions. These combine a glucuronic acid, sulfuric acid, acetic acid, or an amino acid with the drug molecule to make it more polar. The highly polar drugs can then be excreted by the kidney.

RENAL EXCRETION

> Renal elimination of drugs involves three physiologic processes: glomerular filtration, proximal tubular secretion, and distal tubular reabsorption.

1. *Glomerular filtration:* Free drug flows out of the body and into the urine-to-be as part of the glomerular filtrate. The size of the molecule is the only limiting factor at this step.

2. *Proximal tubular secretion:* Some drugs are actively secreted into the proximal tubule.

3. *Distal tubular reabsorption:* Uncharged drugs may diffuse out of the kidney and escape elimination. Manipulating the pH of the urine may alter this process by changing the ionization of the weak acids and bases. This process was described in Chapter 3 in the context of passive diffusion of drugs across membranes. However, for a drug to be excreted, it needs to be charged so that it is trapped in the urine and can't cross the membrane to sneak back into the body.

> **Reminder:** When the pH is higher than the pK, the unprotonated forms (A^- and B) predominate. When the pH is less than the pK, the protonated forms (HA and BH^+) predominate.

PART II Drugs That Affect the Autonomic Nervous System

CHAPTER 6:   Review of the Autonomic Nervous System   27

CHAPTER 7:   Cholinergic Agonists   35

CHAPTER 8:   Cholinergic Antagonists   40

CHAPTER 9:   Adrenergic Agonists   44

CHAPTER 10:   Adrenergic Antagonists   49

Review of the Autonomic Nervous System

Why Include This Material?

Relevant Anatomy

Synthesis, Storage, Release, and Removal of Transmitters

Receptors

General Rules of Innervation

Presynaptic Receptors

WHY INCLUDE THIS MATERIAL?

Why include a review of the autonomic nervous system in a book on pharmacology? The main reason is that autonomic pharmacology is easiest if you have an understanding of the anatomy and physiology of the autonomic nervous system. Therefore, a quick review of the autonomic nervous system should simplify the pharmacology. In addition, autonomic pharmacology forms a basis for cardiovascular and central nervous system pharmacology. Consequently, learning the autonomics thoroughly will save you time and effort later on.

RELEVANT ANATOMY

The nervous system is divided into two main parts: the central and the peripheral nervous systems. The central nervous system is made up of the brain and spinal cord. The peripheral nervous system contains everything else. The peripheral nervous system is divided into two branches: the somatic and autonomic nervous systems. The somatic nervous system is mainly the motor system that includes all of the nerves to the muscles. The other branch, the autonomic nervous system, is the part we're interested in here.

> The autonomic nervous system is responsible for maintaining the internal environment of the body (homeostasis).

Knowing the role of the autonomic nervous system in homeostasis makes it easy to remember the target organs served by this system. It is clear that the cardiovascular system needs regulation, but the smooth muscle of the gastrointestinal (GI) tract and the various glands throughout the body also need to be constantly monitored. Let's first consider some points that are true about the *entire* autonomic nervous system before we break the system down into parts.

> Within the autonomic nervous system, two neurons are required to reach a target organ: a preganglionic neuron and a postganglionic neuron.

The preganglionic neuron originates in the central nervous system. It forms a synapse with the postganglionic neuron, the cell body of which is located in autonomic ganglia.

> *All* preganglionic neurons release acetylcholine as their transmitter. The acetylcholine binds to nicotinic receptors on the postganglionic cell.

The preceding statement is a general rule. We'll come back to the transmitter and receptors in more detail later.

The autonomic nervous system is divided into the sympathetic and parasympathetic systems (Figure 6–1). The sympathetic system is catabolic, meaning that it burns energy. It is the one involved in the fight-or-flight response. If you remember this, most of the effects of the sympathetic nervous system make sense. The sympathetic nervous system is also called the thoracolumbar system because the ganglia are located lateral to the vertebral column in the thoracic and lumbar regions. In addition, because the ganglia are fixed along the back, the postganglionic fibers can be quite long. Within the sympathetic system, the preganglionic axons form synapses with many postganglionic cells, thus giving this system widespread action. Note that this is consistent with the fight-or-flight response.

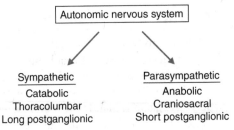

FIGURE 6–1 The two divisions of the autonomic nervous system are illustrated, along with some of the key features of each division.

The parasympathetic system is anabolic, which means that it tries to conserve energy. It is sometimes called the *craniosacral system*. The preganglionic neurons are found in the brainstem and in the sacral region of the spinal cord. In the parasympathetic system, the ganglia are located closer to the target organs (they are not fixed along the vertebral column). Therefore, the preganglionic axons tend to be longer and the postganglionic fibers are shorter. Within the parasympathetic system, one presynaptic axon tends to form a synapse with only one or two post-ganglionic cells, giving the parasympathetic system a more localized action.

> *All* of the parasympathetic postganglionic fibers release acetylcholine. At the target organ acetylcholine interacts with muscarinic receptors.

The keyword here is *all*. More on the muscarinic receptors later.

> *Most* of the sympathetic postganglionic fibers release norepinephrine. At the target organ norepinephrine interacts with a variety of receptors.

The keyword here is *most*. Most of the sympathetic system utilizes norepinephrine (NE), but acetylcholine is also found (in sweat glands). In addition, the adrenal medulla is considered a part of the sympathetic nervous system and it releases epinephrine (EPI, 80%) and NE. Note also that NE is equivalent to nor*adren*aline, and that EPI is equivalent to *adren*aline (hence the term *adren*ergic).

SYNTHESIS, STORAGE, RELEASE, AND REMOVAL OF TRANSMITTERS

The synthesis, storage, release, and removal of transmitters are important because there are drugs that target each of these steps. Let's start with acetylcholine.

> Acetylcholine is synthesized from acetyl coenzyme A (acetyl CoA) and choline. Its action is terminated by acetylcholinesterase.

It is easy to remember the precursors of acetylcholine from the spelling of its name.

Notice that *acetyl* CoA plus *choline* gives you acetylcholine. Likewise, the ending "-esterase" identifies the enzyme that breaks down the acetylcholine.

Now let's turn to NE and its close relative, EPI. It is important to know the pathway for synthesis of these two compounds, at least by name (Figure 6–2).

The rate-limiting step in the synthesis of NE and EPI is the conversion of tyrosine to dopa by tyrosine β-hydroxylase. Although this step is not very important pharmacologically, it seems to appear as an examination question in rather (un)predictable places.

> The effect of NE is terminated predominantly by reuptake into the neuron from which it was released.

NE can also be inactivated by enzymes in the liver (mostly) and brain (some). The degradative enzymes are called COMT (catechol-o-methyltransferase) and MAO (monoamine oxidase). MAO comes in two forms: A and B. COMT,

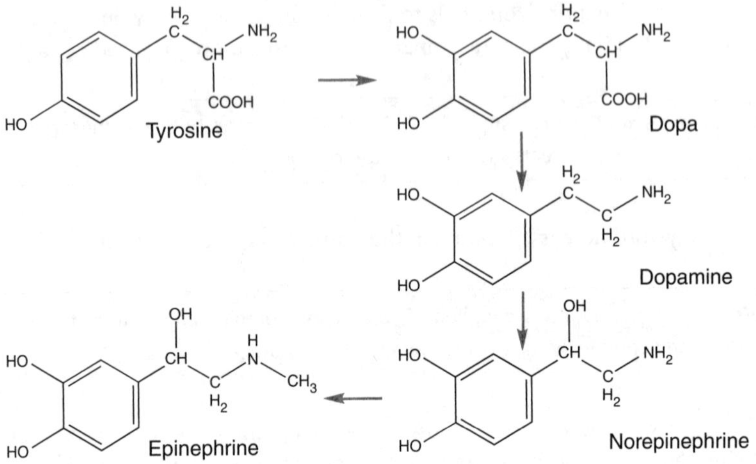

FIGURE 6-2 The synthesis of norepinephrine (NE) and epinephrine (EPI) is illustrated. Note the close relationship between dopamine, NE, and EPI.

particularly in the liver, plays a major role in the metabolism of endogenously released (circulating) and exogenously administered EPI and NE.

Note: You will often hear the term *catecholamine*. This refers to the structure of this group of compounds. They have a catechol group and an amine group, as shown in Figure 6–3.

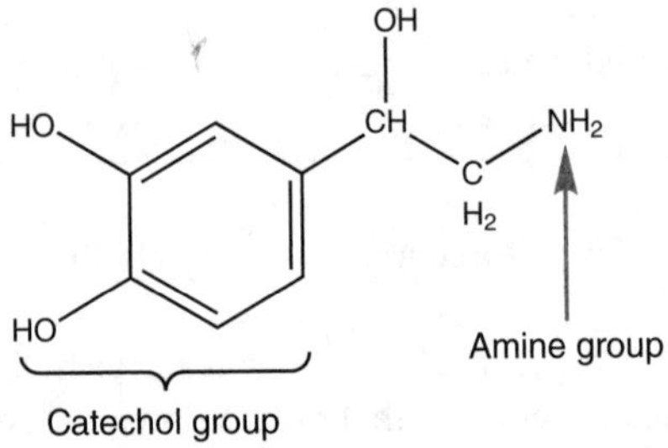

FIGURE 6-3 The general catecholamine structure is illustrated. The catechol group consists of a benzene ring with two hydroxyl groups.

RECEPTORS

There are two major classes of receptors for acetylcholine: muscarinic and nicotinic (Figure 6–4).

There are subtypes of muscarinic receptors (M_1, M_2, and so on), and there are at least two types of nicotinic receptors. Don't attempt to memorize these subtypes until you understand the bigger picture.

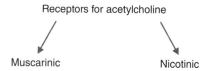

FIGURE 6–4 The types of acetylcholine receptors are illustrated.

> *All* of the parasympathetic postganglionic fibers release acetylcholine. At the target organ the acetylcholine interacts with muscarinic receptors.

This information looks familiar because the same statement was highlighted in an earlier box. These muscarinic receptors are predominantly found in the viscera (GI tract).

> Nicotinic receptors are found at the motor end plate, in all autonomic ganglia, and in the adrenal medulla.

Remember the somatic nervous system that controls movement? It utilizes acetylcholine, and the receptors are all nicotinic. Remember the autonomic ganglia that are present in both the sympathetic and parasympathetic branches? All the preganglionic fibers release acetylcholine, which interacts with nicotinic receptors. Simply add a mental note that the adrenal medulla contains nicotinic receptors.

Now on to the receptors for NE. Students often find these confusing and difficult to learn.

> Receptors for NE are divided into α and β receptors. These receptors are further subdivided into α_1 and α_2, and β_1, β_2, and β_3, respectively.

There are other α and β receptors, but you should focus here on the five subtypes shown in Figure 6–5. These receptors are found in particular target organs. For example, the heart contains mostly β_1 receptors, while β_2 receptors are found

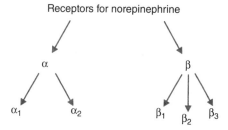

FIGURE 6–5 The subtypes of receptors for norepinephrine (NE) are illustrated.

in blood vessels in the lung and skeletal muscles, and β_3 receptors are found in adipose tissue. This localization of receptor type is the basis of drug therapy. In order to target drug action to the correct organ, drugs have been identified (or designed) that affect only one or two receptor types. This is a very important principle of pharmacology and drug therapy.

GENERAL RULES OF INNERVATION

> Important organs that receive innervation from both the sympathetic and parasympathetic nervous systems include the heart, eye, bronchial smooth muscle, GI tract smooth muscle, and genitourinary tract smooth muscle.

In the preceding box, note the absence of the smooth muscles throughout the vascular system (in the arteries).

When the sympathetic and parasympathetic nervous systems both innervate the same organ system, they have opposite actions. When considering these actions, remember that the sympathetic system (no matter which receptor type is involved) is mediating the fight-or-flight response. For example, both the sympathetic and parasympathetic systems innervate the heart. The sympathetic system increases heart rate and contractility (in order to run faster), while the parasympathetic system decreases heart rate (in order to conserve energy). The one exception to the opposite-effect rule is the salivary glands. Both the sympathetic and parasympathetic systems increase secretion in the salivary glands, but the secretions are of different types.

> In the resting state (not in fight-or-flight situations), most dually innervated organs are controlled by the parasympathetic system.

This state dependence is important when considering drug action. At rest, a drug that blocks the effects of NE (sympathetic) will have little effect, whereas a drug that blocks the effects of acetylcholine at muscarinic receptors (parasympathetic) will have a powerful effect. In contrast, in a situation that is dominated by a fight-or-flight response (such as acute trauma or a highly stressful situation), the blocker of NE will have a greater effect.

Most textbooks include a detailed table of target organs listing the effects of activation of the sympathetic versus the parasympathetic nervous system. Look through the table and first rationalize the sympathetic responses to the fight-or-flight response: the pupils should dilate, the heart rate and contractility should increase, the bronchioles should dilate, the GI tract should shut down (the walls relax and the sphincters contract), the bladder should shut down (the walls relax and the sphincter contracts), blood should be shunted from the GI tract and skin to the muscles, and metabolism should increase the supply of glucose. This makes sense and doesn't need to be memorized.

> Most of the vascular smooth muscle is innervated solely by the sympathetic nervous system. This means that blood pressure and peripheral resistance are controlled by the sympathetic nervous system.

Remember that the vascular smooth muscle is the prime example of a target organ that does not have dual innervation.

> Contraction of the radial muscle (sympathetic innervation) causes dilation, or mydriasis (expected sympathetic response), while contraction of the circular muscle (parasympathetic innervation) causes constriction or miosis (expected parasympathetic response).

The responses in the eye can trip up students. One way to remember these responses is to recognize that the ra*d*ial muscle causes *d*ilation (my*d*riasis) and the *c*ircular muscle causes *c*onstriction (mi*o*sis) (that is, there are no *d*'s in any of the words relating to constriction).

> The heart is the main site for β_1 receptors.

If a drug is specific for β_1 receptors, its main effect will be on the heart. β_1 Receptors are also involved in the release of renin from the kidney.

> Activation of β_2 receptors relaxes smooth muscle.

This is somewhat of a generality, but it is useful to help organize your learning. The smooth muscles that contain the β_2 receptors are found in the blood vessels of skeletal muscles (leading to vasodilation), the GI tract, the bronchial walls, the bladder wall, and the pregnant uterus.

> Activation of α receptors causes contraction or constriction, mostly vasoconstriction.

Again, this simplification is useful to organize your learning. Activation of α receptors contracts blood vessels in the GI tract, contracts the radial muscle in the eye, contracts sphincters in various places, and mediates ejaculation. The last one is the only effect of the sympathetic nervous system that does not fit neatly into fight-or-flight responses.

PRESYNAPTIC RECEPTORS

> Activation of presynaptic α_2 receptors results in feedback inhibition of the release of NE.

Presynaptic receptors are found throughout the central and peripheral nervous systems. The term refers to the receptors found on the presynaptic side of the synapse. These receptors are felt to provide feedback to the neuron about the level of activity at the synapse. Activation or inhibition of these receptors can modulate the release of neurotransmitter from the synapse. In the autonomic nervous system, the presynaptic receptor that gets the most attention is the α_2 receptor. Activation of the presynaptic α_2 receptor decreases the release of NE. In essence when a large amount of NE has been released into the synaptic cleft, the presynaptic receptors are activated to reduce release of even more NE.

> Inhibition of presynaptic α_2 receptors will increase the release of NE.

This is where thinking about presynaptic receptors gets tricky. If we inhibit the presynaptic receptor, the neuron thinks that there is not enough neurotransmitter being released and it increases the release.

Cholinergic Agonists

Organization of Class
Cholinergic Agonists
Cholinesterase Inhibitors

ORGANIZATION OF CLASS

Although I have titled this chapter "Cholinergic Agonists," this chapter, in fact, considers all the drugs that increase activity in cholinergic neurons, sometimes called *cholinomimetics* (because they mimic the action of acetylcholine). There are two main targets of drug action: the postsynaptic receptor and the acetylcholinesterase enzyme, which breaks down acetylcholine.

> Cholinergic agonists have a direct action on the receptor for acetylcholine. Some drugs are specific for the muscarinic receptor; others are specific for the nicotinic receptor.

First, remind yourself where the nicotinic and muscarinic receptors are found:

- Nicotinic receptors are found in autonomic ganglia and at the neuromuscular junction.
- Muscarinic receptors are found on the target organs of the parasympathetic nervous system.

Of course, there are other cholinergic receptors, such as those located in the central nervous system (CNS) and in sweat glands innervated by the sympathetic nervous system. Concentrate on learning the basics and add the others later.

> The cholinesterase inhibitors act by blocking the metabolism of acetylcholine. These drugs effectively increase the concentration of acetylcholine at *all* cholinergic synapses.

The enzyme that is specific for acetylcholine is called *acetylcholinesterase*, and it is found on both the pre- and postsynaptic membranes. There are other cholinesterases (pseudocholinesterase or nonspecific cholinesterase) that are abundant in the liver and can metabolize acetylcholine and drugs with related structures.

The structure and biochemistry of acetylcholinesterase is well studied and an interesting story. Details can be found in most textbooks.

First, review the actions of cholinergic receptor activation.

Activation of Muscarinic Receptors	
Eye	Miosis (constriction of pupil)
Cardiovascular	Decrease in heart rate
Respiratory	Bronchial constriction and increased secretions
Gastrointestinal (GI)	Increased motility, relaxation of sphincters
Genitourinary (GU)	Relaxation of sphincters and bladder wall contraction
Glands	Increased secretions
Activation of Nicotinic Receptors	
Muscle	Fasciculations and weakness

CHOLINERGIC AGONISTS

ESTERS	ALKALOIDS
BETHANECHOL	arecoline
carbachol	muscarine
methacholine	pilocarpine
cevimeline (ring structure)	

These drugs are traditionally divided into two groups: esters of choline that are structurally related to acetylcholine (indicated by "-chol-" in their names), and alkaloids that are not related to acetylcholine and are generally plant derivatives. The only reason that this distinction is important is that the alkaloids, because of their complex structure, are not metabolized by cholinesterases.

The effects of *all* of these agents are exclusively muscarinic.

The preceding statement is sweeping and not entirely true. However, the therapeutically useful drugs in reasonable concentrations are muscarinic. The effects of these drugs were listed earlier, but also can be deduced from your knowledge of the parasympathetic nervous system. The differences between the drugs are related to their resistance to cholinesterase activity and any activity at nicotinic receptors.

BETHANECHOL is used in the treatment of urinary retention.

Of the drugs in this group, bethanechol is the most clinically useful. It is used to treat patients with urinary retention in the postoperative period and in those with a neurogenic bladder. The side effects of these drugs are directly related to their interaction with muscarinic receptors—sweating (increased secretion), salivation, GI distress, and cramps (due to increased motility).

> Nicotine is a direct agonist at nicotinic receptors.

Nicotine is used therapeutically to help patients stop smoking.

CHOLINESTERASE INHIBITORS

These drugs are often divided into two or three groups based on their structure. Words such as *mono-quaternary amine*, *bis-quaternary amine*, *carbamate*, and *organophosphate* appear in many textbooks as names for these subgroups. For our purposes, we'll divide these drugs into two groups: reversible inhibitors, which are water soluble, and irreversible inhibitors (organophosphates), which are lipid soluble.

Reversible Inhibitors		Irreversible Inhibitors
Myasthenia Gravis	**Alzheimer Disease**	**Irreversible Inhibitors**
EDROPHONIUM	DONEPEZIL	diisopropyl fluorophosphate
NEOSTIGMINE	galantamine	echothiophate
PYRIDOSTIGMINE	RIVASTIGMINE	isoflurophate
ambenonium		malathion
demecarium		parathion
physostigmine		sarin
		soman

The reversible inhibitors include the quaternary amines and are the clinically useful drugs. They compete with acetylcholine for the active site on the cholinesterase enzyme. This group includes the drugs with names ending in "-stigmine" and "-nium."

The irreversible inhibitors phosphorylate the enzyme and inactivate it. These cholinesterase inhibitors are widely used as insecticides and are commonly referred to as nerve gases. Because the organophosphates are lipid soluble, they rapidly cross all membranes, including skin and the blood-brain barrier.

> These drugs have all the same actions (and side effects) as the direct-acting drugs (muscarinic). In addition, because they increase the concentration of acetylcholine, they have effects at the neuromuscular junction (nicotinic).

These drugs will cause the same side effects as the direct cholinergic agonists. There is nothing new here. They also affect nicotinic receptors, primarily at the neuromuscular junction. This is the basis of their therapeutic use. They cause fasciculations and weakness in normal people and can improve muscle strength in patients with myasthenia gravis. Myasthenia gravis is an immune disease in which there is loss of acetylcholine receptors at the neuromuscular junction, resulting in weakness and fatigability of skeletal muscle.

These drugs, particularly the organophosphates, can have effects on the cholinergic system in the CNS. The effects range from tremor, anxiety, and restlessness to coma.

> EDROPHONIUM is used in the diagnosis of myasthenia gravis.

Edrophonium is a short-acting cholinesterase inhibitor that is administered intravenously to patients suspected of having myasthenia gravis. If they have myasthenia gravis, the drug will dramatically improve muscle strength. If they do not have myasthenia gravis, what do you think the effects of administration of a cholinesterase inhibitor would be?*

> NEOSTIGMINE, PYRIDOSTIGMINE, and ambenonium are used in the treatment of myasthenia gravis.

These three drugs act in the same way as edrophonium but are longer acting. Therefore, they are used for treatment and not for diagnosis.

> Other uses of the reversible cholinesterase inhibitors: treatment of open-angle glaucoma, treatment of Alzheimer disease, and the reversal of nondepolarizing neuromuscular blockade after surgery.

Studies have shown a deficiency of cholinergic neurons in patients with Alzheimer disease. Cholinesterase inhibitors can increase the concentration of acetylcholine at the remaining cholinergic receptors. None of these agents reverse the disease or ultimately prevent progression. These drugs are able to work because they have more efficacy in the brain than peripherally.

> There are no therapeutic uses for the irreversible cholinesterase inhibitors.

These agents are of interest because of the biochemistry involved in the drug-enzyme interaction and because poisoning with these agents (intentional and unintentional) is common. In 1995, sarin gas was released by a terrorist cult group

---

*These effects could include increased secretions and GI cramping (because of increased motility).

into three different subway lines in Tokyo injuring more than 5500 people. More recently, sarin was used in 2013 during an attack in Syria. There are mnemonics for the effects of organophosphates on muscarinic receptors—SLUDGEM (salivation, lacrimation, urination, defecation, GI motility, emesis, and miosis) or MUDDLES (miosis, urination, diarrhea, diaphoresis, lacrimation, excitation, and salivation). It seems better to just use your knowledge of the physiology of the ANS.

> PRALIDOXIME and ATROPINE are used to treat poisoning with organophosphates.

The organophosphates phosphorylate the cholinesterase enzyme, thus inactivating it. Pralidoxime is able to hydrolyze the phosphate bond and reactivate the enzyme. This works well if the enzyme-phosphate complex has not "aged" (an interesting story). In addition, because pralidoxime does not cross the blood-brain barrier, it is not effective in reversing the CNS effects of the organophosphates. Atropine (a muscarinic antagonist) will block the effects of the excess acetylcholine, but only at the muscarinic receptors. It has no effect at the neuromuscular junction (nicotinic).

Cholinergic Antagonists

Organization of Class
Muscarinic Antagonists
Ganglionic Blockers
Neuromuscular Blockers

ORGANIZATION OF CLASS

The drugs in this group antagonize the effects of acetylcholine. Most of these drugs are antagonists directly at the nicotinic or muscarinic receptor. Some act on the ion channel associated with the nicotinic receptor, and still others block acetylcholine release.

MUSCARINIC ANTAGONISTS

The prototypic muscarinic antagonist is ATROPINE.

In this group of compounds, it is useful to consider a prototype drug and then compare the other drugs with it. The prototype drug for the muscarinic antagonists is atropine.

All of the muscarinic antagonists are competitive antagonists for the binding of acetylcholine to the muscarinic receptor.

These drugs compete with acetylcholine for binding to the muscarinic receptor. They have no intrinsic activity. In other words, in the absence of acetylcholine, they would have no effect.

The effects and side effects of these drugs are opposite of the drugs considered in Chapter 7 (the cholinomimetics)	
Eye	Mydriasis, cycloplegia (blurred vision)
Skin	Reduced sweating, flushing
Gastrointestinal (GI)	Reduced motility and secretions
Cardiovascular	Increased heart rate (high doses)
Respiratory	Bronchial dilation and decreased secretion
Genitourinary (GU)	Urinary retention
Central nervous system (CNS)	Drowsiness, hallucinations, coma

Compare these effects to those listed in the corresponding box in Chapter 7. The important ones to remember are the common side effects of drugs that have anticholinergic properties (many of the CNS drugs); that is, dry eyes, dry mouth, blurred vision, constipation, and urinary retention. If you master the anticholinergic effects now, it will save your considerable effort later.

Many muscarinic antagonists are currently available, and their names do not sound all alike. Some name recognition exercises may be useful here.

Muscarinic Antagonists		
ATROPINE	benztropine	pirenzepine
IPRATROPIUM	cyclopentolate	propantheline
SCOPOLAMINE	darifenacin	solifenacin
	dicyclomine	tolterodine
	fesoterodine	trihexyphenidyl
	glycopyrrolate	tropicamide
	oxybutynin	trospium

Some of these drugs have particular uses. Learn the names of these drugs first and add the others later.

Muscarinic antagonists are used preoperatively to reduce secretions.

SCOPOLAMINE is used to prevent motion sickness.

Scopolamine has an effect on the CNS to reduce motion sickness. It is usually administered using a transdermal patch.

Long-acting anticholinergics are used in the treatment of chronic obstructive pulmonary disease (COPD) to produce bronchodilation.

As you know from Chapter 6, activation of β_2 receptors will result in relaxation of the smooth muscle in the bronchial tree. Thus, β_2 agonists will produce bronchodilation. So will muscarinic antagonists, such as glycopyrrolate and tiotropium. Whether to use a β_2 agonist or a muscarinic antagonist in a particular patient has to do with the underlying pathophysiology of the pulmonary disease and the side-effect profiles of the different bronchodilators.

> Muscarinic antagonists are used for urinary frequency, urgency, and urge incontinence caused by bladder (detrusor) overactivity.

Detrusor overactivity is a common cause of urinary incontinence in elderly patients. As you might expect, these drugs cause dry mouth and constipation.

Other drugs in this group are used to produce mydriasis, treat patients with Parkinson disease and as adjuncts in the treatment of irritable bowel syndrome.

GANGLIONIC BLOCKERS

Ganglionic blockers work by interfering with the postsynaptic action of acetylcholine. They block the action of acetylcholine at the nicotinic receptor of all autonomic ganglia. These drugs are very rarely used clinically.

NEUROMUSCULAR BLOCKERS

These drugs are a little out of place in a section on drugs affecting the autonomic nervous system. However, because they block the effects of acetylcholine by interacting with nicotinic receptors, we'll consider them here.

> The competitive neuromuscular blocking drugs are used to produce skeletal muscle relaxation.

All of these drugs bind to all nicotinic receptors (at the neuromuscular junction and autonomic ganglia) and some actually bind muscarinic receptors to a small extent. The neuromuscular blockers act relatively selectively at the nicotinic receptor at the neuromuscular junction. They vary in their potency and in their duration of action.

The drugs are classified as depolarizing or nondepolarizing blockers based on their mechanism of action. The depolarizing blocker binds to the receptor and opens the ion channel, resulting in depolarization of the end plate (hence its name). The nondepolarizing blockers bind to the receptor, but do not open the ion channel.

The effects of all of these drugs can be reversed by administration of a cholinesterase inhibitor (to increase the amount of acetylcholine available to compete with the receptor blocker). A muscarinic antagonist is often administered at the same time. Can you rationalize why? Hint: You only want to increase the acetylcholine concentration at the neuromuscular junction, which is nicotinic, but the cholinesterase inhibitor works everywhere. Further down on your trivia list is sugammadex. Sugammadex can also be used to reverse the neuromuscular blockade after use of vecuronium or rocuronium (nondepolarizing blockers). It works by forming complexes with rocuronium or vecuronium preventing their binding to the nicotinic receptors.

> SUCCINYLCHOLINE is the <u>only</u> depolarizing neuromuscular blocker.

To make things simpler, there is only one depolarizing agent that you need to know: succinylcholine. Succinylcholine has a brief action, and its use has been associated with malignant hyperthermia, which can be *fatal*.

Now, let's move on to the nondepolarizing blockers. There are several of these.

Nondepolarizing Blockers	
d-TUBOCURARINE	mivacurium
atracurium	PANCURONIUM
cisatracurium	pipecuronium
doxacurium	rocuronium
gallamine	vecuronium
metocurine iodide	

Notice that most of the drug names contain the letters "-cur-," often -curonium or -curium. This should make it easier to recognize the drugs in this group when you see them.

The neuromuscular junction (and other cholinergic synapses) can also be blocked by drugs that block the release of acetylcholine.

> Botulinum toxin blocks the release of acetylcholine at all cholinergic synapses.

We usually think of botulinum toxin as a very potent poison that causes botulism. However, it has found a therapeutic use in the treatment of prolonged muscle spasm and for excessive sweating. A small amount of the toxin is injected directly into a muscle fiber paralyzing the muscle, or in the skin blocking stimulation of the sweat glands. Botulinum toxin is also being used to "treat" wrinkles.

> DANTROLENE is used to treat malignant hyperthermia.

That was a short aside. There was no good place to put dantrolene, and you need to know its name and use. You may also wish to learn its mechanism of action. It interferes with the release of calcium from the sarcoplasmic reticulum in skeletal muscle.

CHAPTER

9

Adrenergic Agonists

Organization of Class
Direct-Acting Agonists
Dopamine
Indirect-Acting Agents
Cardiovascular Effects of Norepinephrine and Epinephrine

ORGANIZATION OF CLASS

This chapter considers the drugs that mimic the effects of adrenergic nerve stimulation (or stimulation of the adrenal medulla). In other words, these compounds mimic the effects of norepinephrine or epinephrine. These drugs are sometimes referred to as *adrenomimetics* or *sympathomimetics*. Remember that the actions of the sympathetic nervous system are mediated through α and β receptors.

Remember that:

α_1 = most vascular smooth muscle; agonists contract

β_1 = heart; agonists increase rate

β_2 = respiratory and uterine smooth muscle; agonists relax

There are other effects of sympathetic stimulation, but the three listed in the preceding box are the most important.

The adrenergic agonists are often divided into direct- and indirect-acting agonists. This is a useful distinction for a number of reasons. The direct-acting drugs bind to receptors, so specificity of action is a possibility. The indirect-acting drugs do not bind to specific receptors but act by releasing stored norepinephrine. This means that their actions are nonspecific.

The drugs are also sometimes divided into catecholamines and noncatecholamines. This is yet another division based on structure (and our focus here is not on structures). However, this distinction is useful for one concept. Do you remember from Chapter 6 that norepinephrine is metabolized by catechol-o-methyltransferase (COMT) and monoamine oxidase (MAO)? Well, the other catecholamines are also metabolized by these enzymes; however, the noncatecholamines are not.

DIRECT-ACTING AGONISTS

The focus here is to learn the specificity of the drugs for their receptor targets. If you know the effect of stimulation of the target receptors, you can deduce the drug actions and adverse effects.

> Only EPINEPHRINE and NOREPINEPHRINE activate both α and β receptors.

Although this is an oversimplification, it provides a useful starting point. The rest of the direct-acting drugs act on either α or β receptors (Figure 9–1). Epinephrine has approximately equal effects at all α and β receptors. Notably, it has approximately equal effects at β_1 and β_2 receptors.

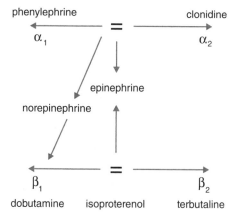

FIGURE 9–1 A classification of adrenergic agonists is presented. Affinity for α receptors is shown at the top of the diagram and affinity for β receptors at the bottom. Epinephrine and norepinephrine have affinity for both α and β receptors and are, therefore, placed in the middle.

Epinephrine has a number of uses, including the treatment of allergic reactions and shock, the control of localized bleeding, and the prolongation of the action of local anesthetics.

> NOREPINEPHRINE has a relatively low affinity for β_2 receptors.

Norepinephrine activates both α and β receptors but activates β_1 receptors more than β_2 receptors. Because of its relatively low affinity for β_2 receptors, norepinephrine is not as useful in the treatment of bronchospasm as epinephrine. Why? Because the smooth muscle of the bronchioles is relaxed by activation of β_2 receptors.

Now let's move on to consider the α- and β-specific drugs. The α-specific drugs are easier, so let's begin with them.

Drug	Receptor Effect	Clinical Effect
PHENYLEPHRINE	α_1 agonist	Nasal decongestant
CLONIDINE	α_2 agonist	Decreases blood pressure through a central action

The main effect of α_1 stimulation (with an agonist such as phenylephrine) is vasoconstriction. Local application of a vasoconstrictor to the nasal passages decreases blood flow locally and decreases secretions, thus acting as a nasal decongestant. The action of clonidine is more complex. It activates α_2 receptors in the central nervous system to decrease sympathetic stimulation to the heart and activates presynaptic α_2 receptors on peripheral nerve endings to inhibit the release of norepinephrine.

Drug	Receptor Effect	Clinical Effect
DOBUTAMINE	β_1 agonist	Increases heart rate and cardiac output
ISOPROTERENOL	$\beta_1 = \beta_2$ agonist	
ALBUTEROL	β_2 agonist	Relieves bronchoconstriction
TERBUTALINE		
metaproterenol		
mirabegron/vibegron	β_3 agonist	Treatment of overactive bladder in adults

Basically, the affinity of these drugs for receptors falls on a spectrum from β_1 to β_2 (see Figure 9–1). Dobutamine is closer to the β_1 end of the spectrum; terbutaline and its relatives are closer to the β_2 end. Isoproterenol falls in the middle of the spectrum. The action of dobutamine is actually quite complex and worth reading about.

There are now relatively specific β_3 agonists that are used in the treatment of overactive bladder in adults with symptoms of urge urinary incontinence, urgency and urinary frequency. Activation of β_3 receptors results in relaxation of the detrusor muscle in the bladder and increases bladder capacity.

DOPAMINE

Dopamine is a catecholamine by structure and is a precursor to norepinephrine (see Figure 6–2). Dopamine receptors are located throughout the body and in the central nervous system. The effects of dopamine are dose-dependent. At low doses, dopamine is an agonist at dopamine receptors. At high doses dopamine acts much like norepinephrine. It is worthwhile here to review the section on dopamine in your textbook.

> At low doses, DOPAMINE causes renal and coronary vasodilation. It also activates β_1 receptors in the heart.

In the treatment of shock, dopamine increases heart rate and cardiac output while simultaneously dilating the renal and coronary arteries. The action of dopamine in the renal vascular bed is useful in attempts to preserve renal blood flow and renal function in the presence of overall decreased tissue perfusion (shock).

INDIRECT-ACTING AGENTS

> The indirect-acting sympathomimetic agents act by releasing previously stored norepinephrine.

Because these drugs act by releasing stored norepinephrine, their effects are widespread and nonspecific. Ephedrine and phenylpropanolamine are nasal decongestants. Phenylpropanolamine has also been used as an appetite suppressant. Don't worry if you can't remember these drugs. Be careful, however, not to confuse phenylephrine (the specific α_1 agonist) with these two similarly named indirect agents.

There is also a prodrug of norepinephrine available (droxidopa). It is metabolized by dopa decarboxylase to norepinephrine and has all the effects of norepinephrine. Droxidopa is used to treat neurogenic orthostatic hypotension.

> AMPHETAMINE and its relatives, dexmethylphenidate and methylphenidate, are central nervous system stimulants used to treat attention deficit hyperactivity disorder in children.

Amphetamine and its other relatives are indirect-acting sympathomimetics that have been abused because of their psychostimulant abilities. There are quite a number of formulations of amphetamine producing differing durations of action and abuse potential. Methylphenidate has been used to treat narcolepsy, but newer drugs, modafinil and armodafinil, have less abuse potential. The mechanism of action of modafinil is not understood.

CARDIOVASCULAR EFFECTS OF NOREPINEPHRINE AND EPINEPHRINE

Before we leave the adrenergic activators, it is useful to consider the intersection of physiology and pharmacology in the cardiovascular actions of epinephrine and norepinephrine.. Some textbooks will also consider dopamine in this context. If your book does include dopamine, be sure to note the dose(s) of dopamine that the book illustrates. Consider the effects of these agents on heart rate, cardiac output, total peripheral resistance, and mean arterial pressure. If you find these effects easy enough to remember, add their effects on systolic and diastolic blood pressure.

> Norepinephrine increases total peripheral resistance and mean arterial pressure.

Through stimulation of α receptors, norepinephrine causes constriction of all major vascular beds. This, in turn, causes an increase in resistance and pressure. The increase in blood pressure causes a reflex increase in parasympathetic output to the heart, which acts to slow the heart down. Therefore, heart rate often decreases after administration of norepinephrine despite direct activation of β_1 receptors.

> Epinephrine predominantly affects the heart through β_1 receptors, causing an increase in heart rate and cardiac output.

Although epinephrine activates all α and β receptors; if given systemically, its effects are predominated by effects on the heart. It increases heart rate, stroke volume, and cardiac output. The effects of epinephrine on blood pressure and peripheral resistance are dose dependent. At low doses, there is a fall in peripheral resistance because of vasodilation in the skeletal muscle beds (β_2 effect). At higher doses, there is some vasoconstriction (α_1) balancing the vasodilation (β_2), resulting in little or no change in peripheral resistance. At even higher doses, the vasoconstriction (α_1) will predominate, resulting in an increase in peripheral resistance and blood pressure.

Find graphs of these changes in your textbook and make sure that you understand them.

Adrenergic Antagonists

Organization of Class
Central Blockers
α-Blockers
β-Blockers
Mixed α- and β-Blockers

ORGANIZATION OF CLASS

The effects of the sympathetic nervous system can be blocked either by decreasing sympathetic outflow from the brain, suppressing release of norepinephrine from terminals, or by blocking postsynaptic receptors. Adrenergic antagonists reduce the effectiveness of sympathetic nerve stimulation and the effects of exogenously applied agonists, such as isoproterenol. Most often the receptor antagonists are divided into α-receptor antagonists and β-receptor antagonists. This classification will work for us also.

CENTRAL BLOCKERS

At this point we are finally ready for a short discussion of α_2-receptor agonists. Yes, I did write agonists, not antagonists—and in a chapter on antagonists.

> α_2 Agonists reduce sympathetic nerve activity and are used to treat hypertension.

α_2-Receptor activation inhibits both sympathetic output from the brain and release of norepinephrine from nerve terminals. We have already listed one of these drugs—clonidine. There are others: dexmedetomidine, guanabenz, guanfacine, and tizanidine. α-Methyldopa is metabolized to α-methylnorepinephrine, which is also an α_2 agonist. Because the α_2 agonists reduce the output from the brain to the sympathetic nervous system, they have found a use in the treatment of hypertension. Tizanidine is used for in the treatment of spasticity, and dexmedetomidine is used for sedation.

α-BLOCKERS

Many compounds possess some α-blocking activity in addition to their primary action. For example, the antipsychotics have α-antagonist properties. In the case of the antipsychotics, these actions are considered side effects. The drugs that we will consider here have their primary action as α antagonists.

> Most of the α antagonists allow vasodilation and, thus, decrease blood pressure.

Remember that α-receptor activation results in vasoconstriction. It should follow that α-receptor blockade will produce vasodilation. This is particularly true when the sympathetic nervous system is firing. For example, the sympathetic nervous system is more active in maintaining blood pressure when a person is standing than when lying down. This is why α-blockade results in a greater decrease in blood pressure when someone stands. This effect is called postural hypotension.

> The side effects of the α-blockers are directly related to their α-blocking activity.

For the most part, the side effects of the α-blockers are intuitive. The most common of these effects are postural hypotension and reflex tachycardia.

In Chapter 9, we briefly reviewed the subtypes of α receptors. You could probably have guessed that there are drugs that are specific antagonists for the α_1 receptor and others that are specific for the α_2 receptor (Figure 10–1). As shown in Figure 10–1, phentolamine and tolazoline are about equal in effectiveness at α_1 and α_2 receptors, whereas phenoxybenzamine is a much more effective α_1- than α_2-blocker. The rest of the drugs listed in Figure 10–1 are selective for the α_1 receptor. Notice that the names in this latter group all end in "-azosin."

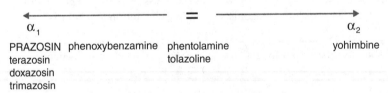

FIGURE 10–1 The relative affinities of various antagonists for the α receptor are schematized.

> TAMSULOSIN and silodosin are specific antagonists of the α_{1A} receptor and are used in the symptomatic treatment of benign prostatic hypertrophy.

Because α_1 receptors mediate contraction in the genitourinary system, α_1 antagonists, such as alfuzosin, can cause the smooth muscle in the bladder neck and prostate to relax and improve urine flow in patients with benign prostatic hypertrophy. Evidence suggests that the subtype of α_1 receptor present in the genitourinary tract is the α_{1A} receptor. Antagonism of this specific receptor reduces the cardiovascular side effects, particularly the orthostatic hypotension.

> All of the α-blockers are reversible inhibitors of the α receptor, except phenoxybenzamine, which is irreversible and used in the treatment of pheochromocytomas.

> The "-azosins," such as PRAZOSIN, are used in the treatment of hypertension.

Because of their specificity for α_1 receptors, prazosin and its relatives (terazosin, doxazosin, and trimazosin) have fewer side effects.

Yohimbine is a selective antagonist at α_2 receptors. It has no clinical role.

β-BLOCKERS

To begin, remind yourself of the localization and action of the β receptors. β_1 Receptors are found in the heart, and their activation leads to an increase in heart rate and contractility. β_2 Receptors are found in smooth muscle of the respiratory tract, the uterus, and blood vessels. Their activation leads to relaxation of the smooth muscle.

> Remember that:
>
> β_1 = heart; antagonists decrease rate
>
> β_2 = smooth muscle; antagonists contract
>
> This latter effect translates into bronchial constriction, which may be dangerous in asthmatics.

The actions of β-blockers on blood pressure are complex. Remember that α receptors control most of the vascular smooth muscle in an unopposed fashion. Chronic administration of β-blockers will, however, decrease blood pressure in people with high blood pressure. The mechanism is not fully understood.

> The β-blockers have widespread use in the management of cardiac arrhythmias, angina, and hypertension (see Part III).

β-Blockers are also used in the treatment of hyperthyroidism, glaucoma, migraines, and anxiety.

> β-Blockers should be used with caution in diabetics.

Recall that the metabolic effects of sympathetic stimulation (glycogenolysis, gluconeogenesis, lipolysis) are mediated by β receptors. In response to hypoglycemia (low blood glucose) the sympathetic nervous system stimulates an increase in blood glucose through β receptors. Blocking this response with a β-blocker will cause the blood glucose to remain low. In addition, the reflex increase in heart rate that occurs in response to hypoglycemia is also blocked by β-blockers. Many diabetics can detect a drop in blood glucose by the reflex increase in heart rate. If you are giving them β-blockers, they lose this early warning sign.

> β_1 Selective antagonists are often referred to as cardioselective.

Most of the β receptors in the heart are β_1 receptors. For this reason, drugs that are selective for the β_1 receptor are referred to as cardioselective.

Nonselective	β_1-Selective
PROPRANOLOL	acebutolol
carteolol	ATENOLOL
levobunolol	betaxolol
nadolol	bisoprolol
penbutolol	esmolol
pindolol	METOPROLOL
timolol	

Looking at the names only, there is no good way to distinguish the cardioselective drugs from the others, and it is not really important at this stage to know which they are. On the bright side, it's easy to recognize the "-olol" ending in the names of the β-blockers.

Besides their receptor selectivity, these drugs vary in duration of action and metabolism.

> The adverse effects of these drugs are, for the most part, directly related to their β-blocking abilities.

The β-blockers can cause bronchoconstriction, decreased heart rate, and cardiac output. Any of these actions could be considered side effects.

> Some β-blockers are said to have intrinsic sympathomimetic activity. This means they have partial agonist activity, even though they are classified as β-blockers.

Students often find the idea of intrinsic sympathomimetic activity confusing. These drugs bind well to the β receptor. In the absence of lots of competing catecholamines, they activate the receptor a little bit. When there are lots of catecholamines, however, these drugs block the receptor from further activation by the catecholamines. Thus, it may be best to simply think of them as partial agonists with high affinity for the receptor. However, they are classified under β-blockers. At this point, it is important to know that some β-blockers have intrinsic sympathomimetic activity, but it is not necessary to memorize the names.

MIXED α- AND β-BLOCKERS

Several drugs are classified as both α- and β-blockers. The oldest of these is labetalol.

First, notice that labetalol does not end in "-olol," but in "-alol." Use this clue to remember that labetalol is different from the other β-blockers.

> Labetalol has both α- and β-blocking activity.

Because of the ratio of β-to-α activity, labetalol is most often listed as a β-blocker with some α-blocking activity. It is nonselective at the β receptor but is specific for α_1 receptors. Its effects are rather complex but make for interesting reading. You can use the mechanism of action of this drug to test your understanding of the adrenergic receptors and their actions.

Another mixed antagonist is CARVEDILOL. It is listed as a nonselective β–blocker with no intrinsic sympathomimetic activity and as an α_1-blocker. This makes it very similar to labetalol. As with labetalol, notice how its spelling (the "-ilol" ending) provides a clue to the different action of this drug.

PART III Drugs That Affect the Cardiovascular System

CHAPTER 11: Diuretics   57

CHAPTER 12: RAS (ACE Inhibitors and ARBs) and
             CCB (Calcium Channel Blockers)   62

CHAPTER 13: Antihypertensives Drugs   66

CHAPTER 14: Drugs Used in Ischemic Heart Disease
             and Congestive Heart Failure   71

CHAPTER 15: Antiarrhythmic Drugs   77

CHAPTER 16: Drugs That Affect Blood   83

CHAPTER 17: Lipid-Lowering Drugs   90

Diuretics

Organization of Class
Diuretics
    Inhibitors of the Na^+-K^+-$2Cl^-$ Symport or Loop Diuretics
    Inhibitors of Na^+/Cl^- Symport or Thiazide Diuretics
    Inhibitors of Renal Epithelial Na^+ Channels or K^+-Sparing Diuretics
    Mineralocorticoid Receptor Antagonists or Aldosterone Antagonists
    Inhibitors of Carbonic Anhydrase
    Osmotic Diuretics
    Inhibitor of Nonspecific Cation Channel or Natriuretic Peptides—Nesiritide

ORGANIZATION OF CLASS

This is a very good time for some review of renal physiology. Remember that the kidney filters the extracellular fluid and the renal nephrons precisely regulate the fluid volume of the body and its electrolyte content via processes of secretion and reabsorption. Disease states such as hypertension, heart failure, renal failure, nephrotic syndrome, and cirrhosis may disrupt this balance.

DIURETICS

Diuretics are drugs that increase the rate of urine flow. Clinically useful diuretics also increase the rate of Na^+ excretion (natriuresis) and of an accompanying anion, usually Cl^-. Most clinical applications of diuretics are directed toward reducing extracellular fluid volume by decreasing total-body NaCl content. Diuretics play an important role in the management of cardiovascular disease and are often used in combination with other classes of drugs.

Name recognition is extremely important with these drugs. Students have missed an exam (or board) question because they didn't recognize a drug (for example) as a potassium-sparing diuretic. This recognition is made more difficult by the fact that the names of these drugs do not have similar endings (or beginnings).

There are three main groups of diuretics and then several others—classified by their mechanisms of action and (often grouped) according to their structural class.

1. Inhibitors of Na^+-K^+-$2Cl^-$ symport: loop diuretics
2. Inhibitors of Na^+/Cl^- symport: thiazide-type diuretics
3. Inhibitors of renal epithelial Na^+ channels: K^+-sparing diuretics
4. Mineralocorticoid receptor antagonists (MRA): Aldosterone antagonists, K^+-sparing
5. Inhibitors of carbonic anhydrase
6. Osmotic diuretics
7. Inhibitors of nonspecific cation channel: natriuretic peptides—nesiritide

Note that groups 3 and 4 are referred to as *potassium-sparing*. This tells you that the other groups cause a *loss* of potassium. You now know a major side effect of diuretics. Next consider the name *loop* diuretics. If you have to guess the site of action of these drugs, what would you guess? I am sure you said the loop of Henle. So you see, you already know the site of action of this group.

INHIBITORS OF THE NA$^+$-K$^+$-2CL$^-$ SYMPORT OR LOOP DIURETICS

FUROSEMIDE	torsemide
BUMETANIDE	azosemide
ETHACRYNIC ACID	piretanide

> The loop diuretics inhibit the symporter in the loop of Henle that moves Na^+, K^+, and Cl^- into the cells and out of the urine.

Their action in the loop of Henle gives the loop diuretics their name. Now you simply need to remember that these drugs inhibit ion reabsorption, which increases ion concentration in the urine—taking additional water with it. Not surprisingly, this results in urinary excretion of Na^+ and Cl^-, but also Ca^{2+}, Mg^{2+}, and K^+.

> The major side effect of the loop diuretics is hypokalemia.

Again, there is nothing new in this statement. The loop diuretics are more potent than the thiazide diuretics. They are the preferred diuretics in patients with low glomerular filtration rates. They can cause a host of metabolic abnormalities, the most common being hypokalemia (low K^+). Dehydration can also be a problem. Finally, they can increase the toxicity of drugs that cause damage to the ear (ototoxicity) and to the kidney (nephrotoxicity). Loop diuretics can cause asymptomatic hyperuricemia. The loss of fluid with use of loop diuretics will stimulate renin release (remember your physiology!!).

> The loop diuretics are used to reduce acute pulmonary edema and in chronic congestive heart failure.

Loop diuretics can be given intravenously for an immediate response and can also be given orally. Loop diuretics are used in the treatment of pulmonary edema because of their potency and rapid onset of action. Loop diuretics are also useful in treating patients with hypertension caused by renal insufficiency.

INHIBITORS OF NA⁺/CL⁻ SYMPORT OR THIAZIDE DIURETICS

Thiazide Diuretics	Thiazide-like Diuretics
bendroflumethiazide	chlorthalidone
chlorothiazide	indapamide
HYDROCHLOROTHIAZIDE	metolazone
methychlothiazide	

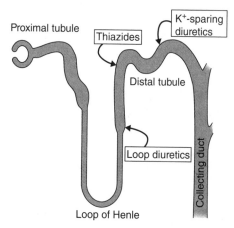

FIGURE 11–1 The location of action of the different classes of diuretics is illustrated here. The loop diuretics act in the ascending loop of Henle. The thiazide diuretics and potassium (K)-sparing diuretics act in the distal tubule.

> The thiazide diuretics inhibit sodium and chloride reabsorption in the thick ascending loop of Henle and early distal tubule (Figure 11–1).

These extra ions in the urine take water with them, thus increasing urine volume. The effect on urine volume is modest because most of the filtered Na^+ was already reabsorbed before the distal tubule. The diuretic effect of thiazides is not solely responsible for their effectiveness as antihypertensives.

All thiazide diuretics are secreted into the urine by the organic acid secretory system in competition with the secretion of uric acid. Because of this, use of thiazide diuretics may result in an increase in serum uric acid levels.

> The thiazide diuretics can cause hypokalemia.

Although adverse effects are uncommon, thiazide diuretics can cause depletion of the extracellular volume, hypotension, decreases in serum Na^+, K^+, Cl^-, Mg^{2+}, and increases in serum Ca^{2+}. They can also decrease glucose tolerance. The hypokalemia can lead to muscle cramps and arrhythmias. The antihypertensive effect of thiazide diuretics may take 4 to 6 weeks.

The most common use of thiazide diuretics is in the treatment of hypertension. They are also used in the treatment of edema associated with heart, liver, and kidney diseases.

INHIBITORS OF RENAL EPITHELIAL NA$^+$ CHANNELS OR K$^+$-SPARING DIURETICS

TRIAMTERENE	AMILORIDE

Mostly used in combination with thiazide or loop diuretics in the treatment of edema and hypertension. Can cause hyperkalemia.

MINERALOCORTICOID RECEPTOR ANTAGONISTS OR ALDOSTERONE ANTAGONISTS

Normally, binding of aldosterone to its cytosolic receptor causes salt and water retention and increases K^+ and H^+ excretion. Thus, it makes sense that blocking these receptors will result in salt and water excretion and a decrease in K^+ excretion.

Used in combination for the treatment of edema and hypertension. Because SPIRONOLACTONE binds to progesterone and androgen receptors, it can cause endocrine abnormalities such as gynecomastia, impotence, and menstrual irregularities.

INHIBITORS OF CARBONIC ANHYDRASE

Carbonic anhydrase is an enzyme that takes carbon dioxide, adds water, and forms bicarbonate and hydrogen ions. It is found throughout the body. In the kidney, it contributes to $NaHCO_3$ reabsorption and acid secretion. Inhibition of carbonic anhydrase reduces the reabsorption of $NaHCO_3$ in the proximal tubule leading to an increase in urinary pH and development of metabolic acidosis.

Carbonic anhydrase inhibitors are used for glaucoma, absence seizures (ACETAZOLAMIDE, CH 23), and in the prevention and treatment of mountain sickness (ACETAZOLAMIDE)

OSMOTIC DIURETICS

Osmotic diuretics are molecules that distribute in the extracellular fluid and add to the osmolality. This results in water moving out of the intracellular spaces to try and reduce the extracellular osmolality. In the proximal tubule, osmotic diuretics act as non-reabsorbable molecules that limit the movement of water thus sodium is no longer reabsorbed. Osmotic diuretics will increase urinary excretion of nearly all electrolytes.

> MANNITOL (an osmotic diuretic) is used to control intracranial pressure.

INHIBITOR OF NONSPECIFIC CATION CHANNEL OR NATRIURETIC PEPTIDES—NESIRITIDE

The natriuretic peptides cause an increase in Na^+ excretion, vasodilation, and reduced production of renin and aldosterone. Used intravenously in the management of acutely decompensated congestive heart failure.

12 RAS (ACE Inhibitors and ARBs) and CCB (Calcium Channel Blockers)

Drugs That Interfere with the Renin-Angiotensin System
   Angiotensin-Converting Enzyme Inhibitors
   Angiotensin II Receptor Blockers
   Direct Renin Inhibitor—Aliskiren
Calcium Channel Blockers

DRUGS THAT INTERFERE WITH THE RENIN-ANGIOTENSIN SYSTEM

The renin-angiotensin system plays a central role in the regulation of fluid balance in the body. Before moving on to the drugs that interfere in this system, take a few moments to review the physiology (Figure 12–1). Note that this system utilizes the kidney, liver, lungs, and adrenal glands. In addition, review the roles for renin, angiotensinogen, angiotensin I, and angiotensin II. Who does what and where?

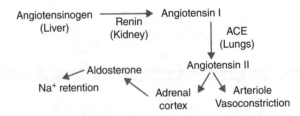

FIGURE 12–1 The renin-angiotensin-aldosterone system.

ANGIOTENSIN-CONVERTING ENZYME INHIBITORS

Angiotensin-converting enzyme (ACE, also known as peptidyldipeptide hydrolase or peptidyl dipeptidase) converts angiotensin I to angiotensin II, which is a potent vasoconstrictor and stimulator of aldosterone secretion. The aldosterone then promotes sodium and water retention and potassium excretion. This leads to an increase in vascular volume and an increase in peripheral vascular resistance.

> Angiotensin-converting enzyme (ACE) inhibitors block the synthesis of angiotensin II.

Blocking the synthesis of angiotensin II leads to a decrease in levels of this circulating vasoconstrictor, which results in a decrease in blood pressure (i.e., afterload). ACE inhibitors also reduce aldosterone secretion, which results in a net water loss (also decreasing afterload).

The currently available ACE inhibitors ("-prils") are listed in the following table. Feel free to add to this list as needed.

ACE Inhibitors	
captopril	moexipril
benazepril	quinapril
ENALAPRIL	ramipril
fosinopril	trandolapril
LISINOPRIL	

ACE inhibitors have several uses, most prominently in the treatment of patients with hypertension (see Chapter 13) and heart failure (see Chapter 14). In hypertensive patients, ACE inhibitors reduce blood pressure while causing little or no change in cardiac output. The antihypertensive effects of the ACE inhibitors are additive with the effects of many other drugs.

These drugs are particularly useful in hypertension that is a result of increased renin levels. Because they do not affect glucose levels, ACE inhibitors are also used in the treatment of hypertension in patients with diabetes. ACE inhibitors have been shown to preserve renal function in patients with nephropathy. The major side effects of these drugs are headache, dizziness, abdominal pain, confusion, renal failure, and impotence. ACE inhibitors can also cause a dry cough thought to be due to bradykinin.

ANGIOTENSIN II RECEPTOR BLOCKERS

These drugs are competitive antagonists of the AT_1 angiotensin receptor.

Angiotensin II Receptor Blockers (ARBs)	
candesartan	olmesartan
eprosartan	telmisartan
LOSARTAN	VALSARTAN
irbesartan	

Notice that, so far, the names of the drugs in the preceding box all end in "-sartan." However, this is no guarantee that new ones under development will retain the "-sartan" ending.

> The angiotensin II receptor blockers (ARBs) are competitive antagonists at the AT_1 angiotensin receptor.

These drugs prevent activation of the angiotensin receptor; hence, their actions are very similar to the actions of ACE inhibitors, which block the formation of angiotensin II. Angiotensin II receptor blockers (ARBs) are as effective in lowering blood pressure and are also cardio- and renal protective with fewer side effects (less cough) than ACE inhibitors.

> ACE inhibitors and ARBs are contraindicated in pregnancy and can cause acute renal failure in patients with bilateral renal artery stenosis.

DIRECT RENIN INHIBITOR—ALISKIREN

Aliskiren is the only currently available renin inhibitor. It competitively inhibits the cleavage of angiotensin I from the precursor angiotensinogen by the enzyme renin. It is used for the treatment of hypertension. It is generally well tolerated, but as with the ACE inhibitors and ARBs, it is not recommended in pregnancy.

CALCIUM CHANNEL BLOCKERS

Before consideration of these drugs, first take a few minutes to review calcium channels—what types/subtypes are found, how they are gated, and other considerations of the physiology. The channels of most interest for pharmacology are the L-type, which are found in cardiac, skeletal, and smooth muscle. Stimulation of these channels results in contraction of the smooth muscle.

> Clinically available calcium channel blockers (CCBs) inhibit the entry of calcium into muscle cells through L-type channels.

There are many calcium channel blockers (CCBs), and the list seems to grow longer every year. These agents differ in pharmacokinetic properties, potency, and selectivity of action. The names of the CCBs all end in "-dipine," "-mil," or "-dil," except diltiazem. Don't confuse diltiazem with diazepam (a benzodiazepine that is used as a sedative; see Chapter 19).

There are two major classes of CCBs:

Dihydropyridine	Nondihydropyridine
AMLODIPINE	VERAPAMIL
felodipine	DILTIAZEM
isradipine	
nifedipine	
nicardipine	

The dihydropyridine CCBs have a relatively greater effect on vascular smooth muscle, so are used for hypertension. The nondihydropyridines have great effects on the heart and are used for arrhythmias.

> The most common side effects of the CCBs (headaches, dizziness, hypotension, etc.) are related to vasodilation.

Remember that the side effects of these drugs are a direct extension of their action. This means you have nothing new to memorize. CCBs are effective in lowering blood pressure and decreasing cardiovascular events in the elderly with isolated systolic hypertension. They can cause cardiac depression, including bradycardia, AV block, cardiac arrest, and heart failure.

CHAPTER

13 Antihypertensive Drugs

Organization of Class
Diuretics
Drugs that Interfere with the Renin-Angiotensin System
    Inhibitors of the Renin-Angiotensin System
    Mineralocorticoid Receptor Antagonists (MRA)
    Direct Renin Inhibitor
Drugs that Decrease Peripheral Vascular Resistance
    Direct Vasodilators
        Calcium Channel Blockers
        Hydralazine, Minoxidil, Nitroprusside
    Sympathetic Nervous System Depressants
        α- and β-Blockers
        Clonidine and Fenoldopam

ORGANIZATION OF CLASS

> Mean arterial pressure = Cardiac output × Peripheral resistance

The preceding equation is a familiar one from physiology. According to this equation, a decrease in either cardiac output or peripheral resistance will decrease blood pressure. Conversely, if high blood pressure, a sustained increase in blood pressure of 140/90 or higher, is present, something must have increased one of the two variables.

A number of factors will increase cardiac output, including increased heart rate, increased contractility, and increased sodium and water retention. Vasoconstriction will increase peripheral resistance. Decreasing one or more of these factors is the goal of antihypertensive therapy.

As you can probably guess, it is easiest to organize the antihypertensive drugs by their mechanism of action. Some of these drugs are also useful in the treatment of angina or heart failure. Many of these drugs have also been covered in Chapters 11 and 12, so only their use in hypertension will be included here.

> I. Diuretics
> II. Drugs that interfere with the renin-angiotensin system, including angiotensin-converting enzyme (ACE) inhibitors and angiotensin II receptor blockers (ARBs)
> III. Drugs that decrease peripheral vascular resistance or cardiac output, including direct vasodilators and drugs that depress the sympathetic nervous system

DIURETICS

Diuretics were covered in more detail in Chapter 11. They play an important role in the management of high blood pressure and are often used in combination with other classes of antihypertensive drugs.

The thiazide diuretics are the most commonly used—sometimes in combination with a K^+-sparing diuretic to reduce K^+ loss. The antihypertensive effect may take 4 to 6 weeks. Hypokalemia is the most common side effect, which may lead to muscle cramps and arrhythmias.

DRUGS THAT INTERFERE WITH THE RENIN-ANGIOTENSIN SYSTEM

The drugs that interfere in the renin-angiotensin system were covered in detail in Chapter 12.

INHIBITORS OF THE RENIN-ANGIOTENSIN SYSTEM

Angiotensin-converting enzyme (ACE) inhibitors and angiotensin II receptor blockers (ARBs) are effective in the treatment of hypertension. They are especially useful in patients with diabetes because they do not affect glucose levels and can slow the progression of renal disease. About 5% of patients will develop a dry cough with ACE inhibitors, but not with ARBs. Both classes of drugs are contraindicated in pregnancy and can take up to 4 weeks to see the full antihypertensive effect.

MINERALOCORTICOID RECEPTOR ANTAGONISTS (MRA)

Spironolactone and eplerenone are antagonists of aldosterone at the mineralocorticoid receptor and can be used to treat hypertension. Remember that aldosterone promotes sodium and water retention and potassium excretion, which leads to an increase in vascular volume and vascular resistance. Blocking the action of the aldosterone receptor will increase urinary excretion of sodium and water. These drugs are used most commonly in heart failure with hypertension and in hyperaldosteronism.

DIRECT RENIN INHIBITOR

Aliskiren is the first direct renin inhibitor available. It binds in the pocket of the renin enzyme blocking its activity. This leads to decreased production of angiotensin I and II and aldosterone.

DRUGS THAT DECREASE PERIPHERAL VASCULAR RESISTANCE

DIRECT VASODILATORS

Calcium Channel Blockers

General issues with calcium channel blockers were covered in Chapter 12. The dihydropyridines can be used as monotherapy or in combination. Calcium channel blockers are effective in lowering blood pressure and decreasing cardiovascular events particularly in the elderly with isolated systolic hypertension.

Hydralazine, Minoxidil, Nitroprusside

There are several other agents that act directly on smooth muscle cells, resulting in vasodilation. For these other drugs, name recognition as vasodilators is the most important thing for you to focus on.

> Hydralazine and minoxidil directly relax arterioles.

The arteriole relaxation results in a decrease in blood pressure that leads to reflex tachycardia and increased cardiac output (not a desirable effect in a patient with limited cardiac reserve). These drugs will also increase plasma renin concentration. The reflex tachycardia can be blocked with β-blockers. Diuretics can be used to counter the sodium and water retention. Hydralazine can induce a lupus syndrome (usually) after at least 6 months of use. Minoxidil is reserved for severe hypertension that does not respond to other medications and should never be used alone.

An aside: Minoxidil causes unwanted hair growth in patients receiving the drug for the treatment of hypertension. The drug is also marketed for topical treatment of baldness (under the trade name Rogaine).

> NITROPRUSSIDE is a vasodilator given by continuous intravenous (IV) infusion. It releases nitric oxide, which activates the cyclic guanosine monophosphate (cGMP) pathway. It releases cyanide when metabolized.

The released nitric oxide increases intracellular cyclic guanosine monophosphate (cGMP), which leads to smooth muscle relaxation. Nitroprusside is used in hypertensive emergencies to rapidly bring down a dangerously high blood pressure. The blood pressure can be controlled with small changes in the intravenous (IV) infusion rate. Use is limited by the release of cyanide and thiocyanate.

SYMPATHETIC NERVOUS SYSTEM DEPRESSANTS

α- and β-Blockers

> The α$_1$ antagonists, such as PRAZOSIN, terazosin, and doxazosin, dilate arteries and veins.

Recall from the discussion of autonomic nervous system drugs that blood vessels are primarily under α receptor control. α Agonists cause vasoconstriction and α antagonists cause vasodilation. The α-blockers can be used to treat hypertension, but they are associated with postural hypotension, particularly after the first dose. The mixed α_1, β_1, and β_2 antagonist, labetalol, dilates blood vessels (α_1) without causing a reflex increase in heart rate (β_1).

β-Blockers prevent sympathetic stimulation of the heart.

β-Blockers have some use in the treatment of hypertension. They decrease heart rate and cardiac output (β_1) and will decrease renin release (β_1). All β-blockers are effective antihypertensives, but the β_1 selective ones have less bronchoconstriction and hypoglycemia (β_2 effects). β-Blockers are used when there is another indication for the use of the β-blocker, such as angina or migraines.

Some β-Blockers Used to Treat Hypertension	
atenolol	β_1 antagonist
bisoprolol	β_1 antagonist
METOPROLOL	β_1 antagonist
carvedilol	β_1 antagonist with α-blocking activity
labetalol	β_1 antagonist with α-blocking activity, used in pregnancy, IV available
nebivolol	β_1 antagonist plus nitric oxide–mediated activity
esmolol	β_1 antagonist plus some sympathomimetic activity
PROPRANOLOL	β_1 and β_2 antagonist
timolol	β_1 and β_2 antagonist

As you can see from the preceding box, both β_1 selective and nonselective blockers have been successfully used in hypertension.

Labetalol is one of the few safe therapeutics in pregnancy.

The mixed α- and β-blockers can also be used in hypertension. Labetalol is available IV and can be used in hypertensive emergencies.

Clonidine and Fenoldopam

Reduction of sympathetic outflow will result in a net decrease in blood pressure. Four drugs are active centrally: clonidine, methyldopa, (or α-methyldopa), guanabenz, and guanfacine. Be sure you know their names and can identify these drugs as centrally active agents that reduce sympathetic outflow.

> CLONIDINE is an α_2 agonist that reduces central sympathetic outflow.

These drugs decrease total peripheral resistance without changing cardiac output. As you might predict, these drugs have no direct effect on the kidney and can be used in patients with renal disease. The side effects of these drugs include drowsiness and dry mouth. There are some differences in the mechanism of action of these compounds, but these differences are too far down on the trivia list to worry about now.

> Fenoldopam, a dopamine agonist, is used for the acute treatment of a hypertensive crisis.

Fenoldopam dilates renal and mesenteric vascular beds by acting as a selective DA_1 receptor agonist.

Drugs Used in Ischemic Heart Disease and Congestive Heart Failure

Ischemic Heart Disease
   Organic Nitrates
Congestive Heart Failure
   Neurohumoral Modulation
   Preload Reduction
   Afterload Reduction
   Enhancement of Contractility—Digoxin
   Heart Rate Reduction
   SGLT2 Inhibition

ISCHEMIC HEART DISEASE

Ischemic heart disease occurs simply when the oxygen demand by the heart exceeds the supply (Figure 14–1). Angina is the primary symptom of ischemic heart disease.

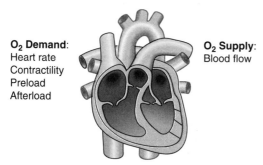

O$_2$ Demand:
Heart rate
Contractility
Preload
Afterload

O$_2$ Supply:
Blood flow

FIGURE 14–1 Ischemic heart disease comes about when one, or more, of the factors that determine oxygen demand by the heart exceeds the blood/oxygen supply to the heart muscle.

To reduce myocardial oxygen demand β-blockers (see Chapters 10 and 13) can be used to decrease heart rate and contractility. Calcium channel blockers (see Chapter 12), particularly verapamil, diltiazem, and amlodipine, reduce systemic vascular resistance, improve coronary and myocardial blood flow, and decrease myocardial contractility. Nitrates (below) will produce venous dilation, which will decrease preload and decrease oxygen demand by the heart. β-Blockers are effective in exertional angina and improving survival in patients who have had a myocardial infarction. Finally, antiplatelet drugs (see Chapter 16), such as aspirin, will prevent thrombus formation in the coronary arteries. Lipid-lowering drugs (see Chapter 17) have been shown to reduce the risk of heart attacks in patients with coronary artery disease.

Unstable angina is treated with nitroglycerin, antiplatelet, and anticoagulant drugs. Finally, acute myocardial infarction is treated with thrombolytic agents (see Chapter 16). Recent guidelines have direct reversible P2Y12 receptor antagonists (ticagrelor and prasugrel) as the primary choice for acute coronary syndrome, which includes myocardial infarction.

ORGANIC NITRATES

> NITROGLYCERIN
>
> isosorbide dinitrate
>
> isosorbide-5-mononitrate

These drugs are sources of nitric oxide (NO), which produces relaxation of vascular smooth muscle leading to vasodilation. The organic nitrates preferentially dilate veins and conductive arteries. The beneficial effect of nitroglycerin appears to come primarily from the reduction in cardiac oxygen demand. The increase in cyclic guanosine monophosphate (cGMP) that results will inhibit platelet function.

> Nitroglycerin is administered under the tongue (sublingually) for rapid onset and to avoid first-pass metabolism.

Hopefully you remember what first-pass metabolism is! Repeated or continuous exposure leads to tolerance. Headache is common and tells the patient that the nitroglycerin is still active. Orthostatic hypotension and tachycardia can also occur.

CONGESTIVE HEART FAILURE

Heart failure occurs when the heart can no longer pump enough blood to meet the demands of the body. Heart failure is a clinical syndrome that represents the final common pathway of multiple cardiac diseases. The most common cause is ischemic heart disease. Other causes include chronic arterial hypertension (HTN), valvular diseases, cardiomyopathies, viral infections and toxins.

Patients with a left ventricular ejection fraction (LVEF) ≤ 40% are considered to have heart failure with reduced ejection fraction (HFrEF). Patients with an LVEF ≥ 50% and symptoms of heart failure are considered to have heart failure with preserved ejection fraction (HFpEF). There has been no medical treatment for patients with HFpEF, but (in 2021) the combination of the neprilysin inhibitor sacubitril and the angiotensin receptor blocker valsartan was approved for the treatment of HFpEF.

The pathophysiology of heart failure involves the heart, vasculature, kidney, and various neurohumoral regulatory circuits. Therefore, the treatment of heart failure is multifactorial with damping of neurohumoral activation, preload and afterload reduction, decreasing heart rate, and increasing cardiac contractility all potentially playing a role.

Drugs That Target the Renin-Angiotensin System			
ACE inhibitor	**ARB**	**β-Blockers**	**Vasodilators**
captopril	candesartan	bisoprolol	Nitrates
enalapril	LOSARTAN	carvedilol	
LISINOPRIL	valsartan	METOPROLOL	**MRA**
fosinopril		nebivolol	eplerenone
perindopril	**ARB-neprilysin inhibitor**		spironolactone
quinapril	sacubitril/valsartan	**Loop diuretics**	
ramipril		bumetanide	**Other**
trandolapril		furosemide	ivabradine
		torsemide	digoxin

All patients with HFrEF should receive one of the drugs that target the renin-angiotensin system (RAS): an angiotensin-converting enzyme (ACE) inhibitor, angiotensin II receptor blocker (ARB), or angiotensin receptor-neprilysin inhibitor (ARNI). They should also receive a β-blocker and, if volume overloaded, a diuretic.

NEUROHUMORAL MODULATION

> Damping neurohumoral activation with ACE inhibitors/ARBs, β-blockers, and mineralo-corticoid receptor antagonists (MRAs) is the main treatment focus in heart failure.

The RAS was covered in more detail in Chapter 12.

> The ACE inhibitors and ARBs reduce hospitalization and prolong survival in patients with heart failure.

Both classes of drugs can result in hypotension. The ACE inhibitors have been shown to reduce long-term remodeling of the heart and its blood vessels. Do not use in patients with bilateral renal artery stenosis (check out the reasoning!). Patients with heart failure taking ACE inhibitors should not take nonsteroidal anti-inflammatory drugs (NSAIDs), which reduce the production of prostaglandins. Can you rationalize this one?

> The combination of sacubitril and valsartan reduces hospitalization for heart failure, in part, by inhibition of neprilysin.

Neprilysin is an enzyme that degrades ANP and BNP (natriuretic peptides). If neprilysin is inhibited, levels of ANP and BNP are elevated. ANP and BNP stimulate membrane guanylyl cyclase, thus elevating levels of cGMP. cGMP is diuretic (kidney) and vasodilatory (vasculature). In addition, in the heart, cGMP is antihypertropic, antifibrotic, and will increase compliance. All of these actions are helpful in heart failure. Sacubitril is a neprilysin inhibitor used in combination with an ARB (valsartan).

Now would be a great time to review the actions of norepinephrine and epinephrine that are mediated through β receptors. As you do that, ask yourself what would be the benefit of using a β-blocker in the treatment of heart failure.

> β-Blockers protect the heart from the consequences of long-term adrenergic stimulation.

Use of β-blockers improves symptoms and clinical outcomes in patients with heart failure. They slow the heart rate, decrease the incidence of arrhythmias, and lower renin levels. It is also thought that they will prolong diastole, thereby improving perfusion of the myocardium.

The mineralocorticoid receptor antagonists (MRAs) reduce the risk of hospitalization and death from heart failure, when added to standard therapy. Remember that aldosterone promotes Na^+ and fluid retention, sympathetic activation, myocardial and vascular fibrosis, baroreceptor dysfunction, and vascular damage. All of these are adverse effects in heart failure, so it makes sense that inhibition of the effects of aldosterone is useful in the treatment of heart failure.

PRELOAD REDUCTION

> In congestive heart failure the heart cannot generate enough force, for the amount of preload, leading to edema in the lungs and periphery. Treatment is diuretics—most often loop diuretics.

Diuretics were covered in detail in Chapter 11. The loop diuretics (bumetanide, furosemide, and torsemide) are more effective in heart failure than thiazide diuretics. The most common adverse effect is hypokalemia. The effect of diuretics on survival is unclear.

AFTERLOAD REDUCTION

> Reduction of afterload should benefit patients with heart failure because the heart pumps against lower pressure. However, use of vasodilators alone results in reflex tachycardia and negative inotropic effects.

ENHANCEMENT OF CONTRACTILITY

The failing heart cannot generate sufficient force to meet the needs of the body. Historically, cardiac glycosides were used to improve contractility. However, their use has decreased significantly because they do not improve life expectancy or cardiac performance.

The cardiac glycosides were originally isolated from the Digitalis purpurea plant; a fact that is reflected in their names—digitalis, digoxin, and digitoxin. The term *digitalis* is a general one that is usually used when referring to the drug digoxin.

> The cardiac glycosides (DIGOXIN and DIGITOXIN) inhibit Na^+–K^+–ATPase.

These drugs inhibit sodium-potassium-ATPase and enhance release of intracellular calcium from the sarcoplasmic reticulum. This increase in intracellular calcium causes an increase in the force of contraction of the myocytes throughout the heart. In addition to their use in chronic heart failure, both digoxin and digitoxin will slow the ventricular rate in atrial flutter or fibrillation by increasing the sensitivity of the atrioventricular (AV) node to vagal stimulation. This makes them antiarrhythmic drugs as well (see Chapter 15).

> The cardiac glycosides have a low therapeutic index.

As noted in Chapter 2, the therapeutic index is the LD_{50} divided by the ED_{50}. A low therapeutic index means that the plasma concentration that causes serious toxicity (i.e., may be fatal) is only slightly higher than the therapeutic dose. The therapeutic index is between 1.6 and 2.5 for the cardiac glycosides. Toxicity of the cardiac glycosides is more common in patients with low serum potassium levels. Use of digoxin is also associated with arrhythmias, which can be life threatening.

HEART RATE REDUCTION

Heart rate is a major contributor to energy needs in the heart. High heart rates in patients with heart failure are associated with a poor prognosis. The heart rate can be kept low pharmacologically with a β-blocker (usually a partial agonist) or by inhibiting the cardiac pacemaker (ivabradine). Ivabradine inhibits the I_f pacemaker channel, resulting in slowing of the heart rate. In some patients with heart failure, it can reduce hospitalization and death.

SGLT2 INHIBITION

We think of the sodium-glucose cotransporter 2 (SGLT2) inhibitors with the treatment of diabetes (see Chapter 41). Well, studies have been done that show a benefit of using dapagliflozin and empagliflozin in the treatment of HFrEF—even in patients without diabetes. When added to standard therapy, patients had fewer hospitalizations and less death if they were given a "-gliflozin".

Antiarrhythmic Drugs

Organization of Class

Class I Drugs (Sodium Channel Blockers)

Class II Drugs (β-Blockers)

Class III Drugs (Potassium Channel Blockers)

Class IV Drugs (Calcium Channel Blockers)

Other Antiarrhythmic Drugs

Drugs That Increase Heart Rate

ORGANIZATION OF CLASS

Arrhythmias, disturbances of the normal rhythm of the heart, occur when the electrical conduction systems malfunction. The malfunction could result in a change in heart rate, rhythm, impulse generation, or electrical conduction. Nonpharmacologic approaches to arrhythmias include the use of pacemakers, implantable defibrillators, and ablation of an aberrant conduction pathway. A number of drugs can cause arrhythmias. Treatment of these arrhythmias is withdrawal of the drug.

To understand the action and classification of the antiarrhythmic drugs, it is first necessary to review the ionic movements during the cardiac action potential (Figure 15–1). It is also good to remember the normal flow of electricity in the heart. What controls the rate? What controls the rhythm? What takes over in emergencies?

The antiarrhythmic agents are classified into four groups according to the part of the cardiac cycle they influence. This is a universal system, but it is not

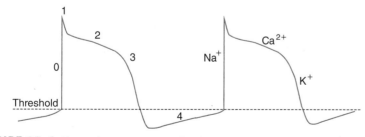

FIGURE 15–1 The cardiac action potential is shown. The action potential has been divided into phases (indicated on the left). The shape of the action potential is determined by the ions that are flowing during that phase (indicated on the right).

entirely accurate. Several drugs have more than one effect, and others do not fall into any of the four categories.

CLASS I DRUGS (SODIUM CHANNEL BLOCKERS)

> The class I drugs are essentially sodium channel blockers.

The class I drugs are characterized by their ability to block sodium entry into the cell during depolarization. This decreases the rate of rise of phase 0 of the action potential (Figure 15–2).

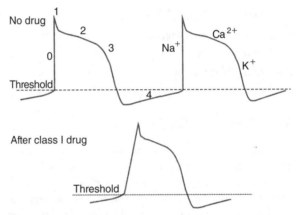

FIGURE 15–2 Class I antiarrhythmics block sodium entry into myocardial cells during depolarization. This decreases the rate of rise of phase 0.

The class I drugs have been further divided into three groups. Class IA drugs slow the rate of rise of phase 0 and prolong the effective refractory period of the ventricle. Class IB drugs have less of an effect on phase 0 but shorten the action potential duration and refractory period of the Purkinje fibers. Class IC drugs have the greatest effect on the early depolarization and have less of an effect on the refractory period of the ventricle.

Class IA Drugs	Class IB Drugs	Class IC Drugs
PROCAINAMIDE	LIDOCAINE	flecainide
QUINIDINE	mexiletine	propafenone
disopyramide	phenytoin	
	tocainide	

Here we have a major stumbling block for pharmacology students. Notice that there appears to be little rhyme or reason in the names given to the class I drugs.

If you have already covered these drugs in class, you may recognize some of the local anesthetics (procainamide and lidocaine). Many of these drug names do look a bit alike, because they end in "-cainide." Name recognition drilling will be most helpful with this group of drugs.

The names and overall mechanism of action are the most important points for you to know about the class I antiarrhythmics. Once you have mastered this information, you can add a few facts about some of the individual agents.

> The class IA drugs are useful in the treatment of atrial and ventricular arrhythmias.

These drugs—quinidine, procainamide, and disopyramide—are all-purpose antiarrhythmics. As you read through the uses and indications for these drugs, focus on the similarities. Later you can go back and consider the differences.

As you might guess from its name, quinidine is related to quinine. Both quinidine and quinine have antimalarial actions (see Chapter 36).

> The class IB drugs (LIDOCAINE is the *drug of choice*) are used for the acute treatment of ventricular arrhythmias (ventricular tachycardia, ventricular fibrillation, and ventricular ectopy).

The class IB drugs are much less effective in treating the atrial (supraventricular) arrhythmias than the class IA drugs.

> The class IC agents are useful in suppressing ventricular arrhythmias.

Flecainide and propafenone are absorbed orally and are used for chronic suppression of ventricular arrhythmias (as opposed to acute treatment, which is the role of the class IB agents).

CLASS II DRUGS (β-BLOCKERS)

> The class II antiarrhythmics are β-blockers.

The mechanism of action of these drugs, in terms of rhythm stabilization, is unknown. Use of the β-blockers results in cardiac membrane stabilization. Conduction through the sinoatrial (SA) and atrioventricular (AV) nodes is slowed, and the refractory period is increased (Figure 15–3). A list of β-blockers is provided in Chapter 10.

> These drugs are particularly useful in suppressing the tachyarrhythmias that result from increased sympathetic activity.

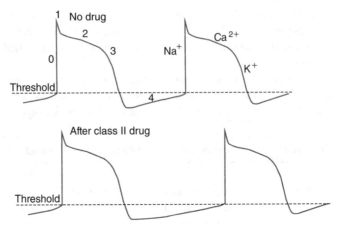

FIGURE 15–3 Class II antiarrhythmics increase the refractory period between action potentials.

CLASS III DRUGS (POTASSIUM CHANNEL BLOCKERS)

> The class III antiarrhythmics prolong the action potential, increase refractoriness and increase contractility. They are sometimes designated as potassium channel blockers.

These drugs show complex pharmacologic properties. They are classified together because they all prolong the duration of the action potential without altering phase 0 depolarization or the resting membrane potential (Figure 15–4).

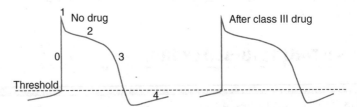

FIGURE 15–4 Class III antiarrhythmics prolong the duration of the action potential without altering phase 0 depolarization or the resting membrane potential.

Class III Drugs	
BRETYLIUM	dofetilide
AMIODARONE	ibutilide
dronedarone	sotalol

It is probably wise to include these drug names in your name recognition list. Note, however, that many books do not include sotalol here. You should check your textbook or lecture notes.

> The class III agents are useful in treating intractable ventricular arrhythmias.

Amiodarone is effective in the treatment and prevention of ventricular fibrillation and ventricular tachycardia. However, dofetilide is used to convert atrial fibrillation and maintain sinus rhythm after cardioversion. So you can see, the general rules don't always apply. Dronedarone is an analogue of amiodarone without the iodine. It appears to be less toxic than amiodarone.

Not all class III drugs block potassium currents. Ibutilide promotes the influx of sodium through slow inward sodium channels, resulting in a prolongation of the action potential. This results in slowing of the heart rate and conduction through the AV node. Ibutilide is indicated for the conversion of atrial fibrillation or flutter to normal sinus rhythm.

CLASS IV DRUGS (CALCIUM CHANNEL BLOCKERS)

> The class IV antiarrhythmics are the calcium channel blockers. These drugs slow conduction through the AV node and increase the effective refractory period in the AV node.

These actions may terminate reentrant arrhythmias that require the AV node for conduction. A list of calcium channel blockers is provided in Chapter 12. Only verapamil and diltiazem block Ca^{+2} channels in cardiac cells at clinically useful doses.

These drugs block the slow inward calcium current during phases 0 and 2 of the cardiac cycle. By slowing the inward calcium current, these drugs slow conduction and prolong the effective refractory period, especially in the AV node.

> The calcium channel blockers are more effective against atrial than ventricular arrhythmias.

The side effects of these drugs are the result of their other actions, such as vasodilation. This should come as no surprise.

OTHER ANTIARRHYTHMIC DRUGS

As previously noted, there are a number of drugs that do not neatly fall into the four classes of antiarrhythmics. Among these other antiarrhythmic drugs are adenosine and the cardiac glycosides (digoxin).

> ADENOSINE is highly effective in terminating paroxysmal supraventricular tachycardia.

Adenosine is given intravenously and has an exceedingly short half-life (in seconds). It depresses AV and sinus node activity. Because the most common form of paroxysmal supraventricular tachycardia involves a reentrant pathway, adenosine is effective in terminating the arrhythmia.

> DIGOXIN is used to control the ventricular rate in atrial fibrillation or flutter.

Digoxin slows conduction through the AV node and increases the refractory period of the AV node. This decreases the number and frequency of impulses that pass from the atria into the ventricles. That's important when the atria are out of control, as in flutter or fibrillation.

DRUGS THAT INCREASE HEART RATE

> Drugs that can be used to increase heart rate include ATROPINE, ISOPROTERENOL, and EPINEPHRINE.

These drugs are used to treat bradycardia. Blocking the parasympathetic system (which tries to slow the heart) with atropine (a muscarinic antagonist) will increase the heart rate. Sympathetic agonists will also increase heart rate by directly stimulating the β receptors in the heart. The increase in heart rate and contractility can worsen ischemia in a patient whose heart is at risk.

Drugs That Affect Blood

Organization of Class

Antiplatelet Agents

Anticoagulants

Thrombolytic Drugs

Phosphodiesterase Inhibitors

Drugs Used in the Treatment of Anemia

Drugs for Sickle Cell Disease

ORGANIZATION OF CLASS

The process of hemostasis consists of three phases: vascular, platelet, and coagulation (Figure 16–1). The fibrinolytic phase that follows prevents the clotting process from spreading out of control beyond the site of injury. It may be helpful at this point to review the hemostatic mechanisms in your physiology textbook.

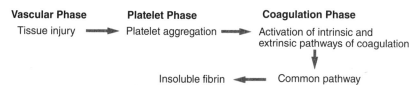

FIGURE 16–1 Hemostasis consists of three phases: vascular, platelet, and coagulation. The end result of these phases is the formation of fibrin.

Platelets respond to tissue injury by adhering to the site of injury; they then release granules containing chemical mediators that promote aggregation. Factors released by platelets and the injured tissue cause activation of the coagulation cascade. This results in the formation of thrombin, which in turn converts fibrinogen to fibrin. The subsequent cross-linking of the fibrin strands stabilizes the clot.

Drugs are available that interfere with the platelet and coagulation phases of the initial response to tissue injury. As we review the drugs that prevent clots and those that lyse clots, the drugs that can function as antidotes will be mentioned. Finally, we'll consider drugs used to treat anemia.

ANTIPLATELET AGENTS

Platelet aggregation inhibitors decrease the formation of chemical signals that promote platelet aggregation. Drugs that inhibit platelet function are administered for the relatively specific *prophylaxis* of arterial thrombosis and during management of heart attacks (myocardial infarction).

> Nonsteroidal anti-inflammatory drugs (NSAIDs), including aspirin, inhibit platelet aggregation and prolong bleeding time.

Antiplatelet Drugs	
NSAIDs, including aspirin	**IIB/IIIA receptor antagonists**
dipyridamole	abciximab
P2Y12 ADP receptor blockers	eptifibatide
ticlopidine	tirofiban
clopidogrel	
prasugrel	
ticagrelor	

Nonsteroidal anti-inflammatory drugs (NSAIDs) will be considered in more detail in Chapter 45. These agents inhibit cyclooxygenase. In platelets, this inhibits the formation of TXA_2 (a thromboxane). TXA_2 is a potent inducer of platelet aggregation. Aspirin acetylates cyclooxygenase-1 (COX-1) effectively inhibiting platelet aggregation for 5 to 7 days.

Dipyridamole decreases platelet adhesion to damaged endothelium but does not alter bleeding time. Dipyridamole inhibits platelet uptake of adenosine. It is usually used in combination with aspirin or warfarin.

Ticlopidine, prasugrel, clopidogrel, and ticagrelor inhibit platelet aggregation and prolong bleeding time. They work by inactivating the platelet P2Y12 (ADP) receptor, thus having a prolonged action. This receptor plays a central role in amplification and stabilization of platelet aggregation (i.e., clot formation).

> Platelet glycoprotein IIb/IIIa receptor antagonists prevent platelet aggregation by blocking the binding of fibrinogen and von Willebrand factor to the glycoprotein IIb/IIIa receptor on the surface of the platelet.

The glycoprotein receptor, known as the IIb/IIIa receptor, is critical for platelet aggregation. Fibrinogen molecules bind to these receptors and form bridges between adjacent platelets, allowing them to aggregate. Abciximab is a monoclonal antibody to the receptor, and eptifibatide and tirofiban are platelet IIb/IIIa receptor antagonists. All of these drugs increase the risk of bleeding, particularly at the site of arterial access.

Finally, vorapaxar inhibits thrombin-induced platelet aggregation by blocking the protease-activated receptor-1 on platelets.

ANTICOAGULANTS

Anticoagulant drugs inhibit the development and enlargement of clots. It should be obvious from the name of the group that the drugs act by interfering with the coagulation phase of hemostasis. These drugs are divided into two to four groups in various books. As the number of available drugs increases, the number of groups will increase.

Anticoagulant Drugs	
Heparin and LMWH	*Thrombin inhibitors*
HEPARIN	hirudin
ardeparin	argatroban
dalteparin	bivalirudin
danaparoid	dabigatran (oral)
enoxaparin	desirudin
tinzaparin	lepirudin
Vitamin K inhibitors (depletors) (oral)	*Direct factor Xa inhibitors* (oral)
warfarin	apixaban
dicumarol	edoxaban
	rivaroxaban
	Others
	fondaparinux
	drotrecogin alfa

> The major side effect of all of the anticoagulants is hemorrhage.

The preceding statement should be intuitive. Anticoagulant therapy provides prophylaxis against venous and arterial thrombosis. These drugs cannot dissolve clots that have already formed, but they may prevent or slow extension of an existing clot. They are useful in preventing deep vein thrombosis and pulmonary embolism. Anticoagulation therapy in patients with atrial fibrillation reduces the risk of systemic embolism and stroke.

> HEPARIN interferes with clotting factor activation in both the intrinsic and extrinsic pathway.

The principal anticoagulant action of heparin is a result of its binding to antithrombin III. Heparin also inactivates factors IIa, IXa, Xa, XIa, XIIa, and XIIIa, and neutralizes tissue thromboplastin (factor III). The low-molecular-weight heparins are oligosaccharides extracted from heparin. These agents have larger anti-Xa to anti-IIa activity ratios than heparin, which permit them to be used at lower doses. In addition, the low-molecular-weight heparins have greater bioavailability after subcutaneous injection and have a longer half-life than heparin.

> PROTAMINE is a specific heparin antagonist that can be used to treat heparin-induced hemorrhage.

Protamines are basic proteins that have a high affinity for the negatively charged heparin. The binding of protamine and heparin is immediate and results in an inert complex.

Before they can participate in the clotting process, several of the protein coagulation factors require vitamin K for their activation. Warfarin interferes with this action of vitamin K, thus delaying activation of new coagulation factors (Figure 16–2). Factors that have already been activated are not affected. This means there is a delay in the onset of action of the vitamin K inhibitors.

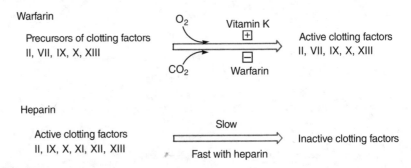

FIGURE 16–2 Diagram of the processes by which warfarin blocks activation of clotting factors and heparin speeds the inactivation of clotting factors.

> Administration of vitamin K can overcome the anticoagulant effects of the warfarin, but the effect takes about 24 hours.

The time it takes for vitamin K to overcome the anticoagulant effects of warfarin is also directly related to the mechanism of action. It takes time to make new coagulation factors.

Several drugs are now available that inhibit factor Xa and are orally active. In addition, they, including apixaban and rivaroxaban, do not require routine monitoring of clotting time. Fondaparinux, a synthetic compound, indirectly inhibits factor Xa by binding to antithrombin. Drotrecogin alfa is a recombinant form of human activated protein C and inhibits factors Va and VIIIa. It may also have anti-inflammatory effects and has been shown to increase survival in patients with sepsis.

> Direct thrombin inhibitors are also effective anticoagulants.

Thrombin plays a number of critical roles in coagulation. The first direct thrombin inhibitor, hirudin, was derived from the medicinal leech. There are now a number of thrombin inhibitors. Urgent reversal of the anticoagulant effect of the orally active direct thrombin inhibitor dabigatran can be achieved with the monoclonal antibody idarucizumab. More are surely in the pipeline.

> There are a large number of drug interactions with the oral anticoagulants.

There are many drugs that both increase and decrease the effect of the oral anticoagulants. It is not possible to memorize them all. The important thing for now is to remember that there are many drug interactions.

THROMBOLYTIC DRUGS

Thrombolytic Drugs	
STREPTOKINASE	reteplase
alteplase	t-PA
anistreplase	tenecteplase
lanoteplase	urokinase

> Anticoagulant and antiplatelet drugs are administered to prevent the formation or extension of clots. Thrombolytic drugs are used to lyse already formed clots.

This is an important distinction for the clinical use of these drugs. Fibrinolysis is the process of breaking down the fibrin that holds the clot together. Fibrinolysis is initiated by the activation of plasminogen to plasmin. The plasmin then catalyzes the degradation of fibrin. The activation of plasminogen is normally initiated by plasminogen activators (straightforward so far?).

> The thrombolytic drugs are plasminogen activators so they catalyze the formation of plasmin.

There are currently two generations of plasminogen activators: first and second. The first-generation drugs (including streptokinase and urokinase) convert all plasminogen to plasmin throughout the plasma. The second-generation drugs (including tissue plasminogen activator or t-PA) selectively activate plasminogen that is bound to fibrin. This is supposed to reduce the side effects of the drug by targeting the site of action.

> Clot dissolution and reperfusion are more likely if therapy is initiated early after clot formation. Clots become more difficult to lyse as they age.

Thrombolytic drugs have been shown to lyse clots in arteries and veins and to reestablish tissue perfusion. They are used in the management of pulmonary embolism, deep vein thrombosis, and arterial thromboembolism. They have proven to be particularly useful in acute heart attacks caused by a clot in a coronary artery.

> The main side effect of the thrombolytic drugs is bleeding.

This statement should not come as a surprise to you.

> STREPTOKINASE is a foreign protein and is antigenic. t-PA is not antigenic.

The antigenicity of streptokinase (a result of its bacterial origin), produces one of the side effects of this drug: an allergic–anaphylactic reaction. Patients may also develop antibodies to streptokinase and inactivate it. These reactions are less likely to occur after t-PA administration, because t-PA is of human origin (produced through recombinant DNA technology).

Recombinant forms of t-PA, including reteplase, alteplase, and lanoteplase, are available. They differ from t-PA in time for onset of action and duration of action.

PHOSPHODIESTERASE INHIBITORS

> Phosphodiesterase III inhibitors (pentoxifylline and cilostazol) are used to treat intermittent claudication.

Intermittent claudication is a symptom of peripheral arterial disease and often causes debilitating pain, aches, and cramps in the legs that reduce a person's ability to walk. These agents target multiple processes related to peripheral circulation, including inhibition of platelet aggregation, and cause vasodilation.

DRUGS USED IN THE TREATMENT OF ANEMIA

Anemia is defined as a plasma hemoglobin level that is below normal. It can reflect decreased numbers of circulating red blood cells or an abnormally low total hemoglobin content. There are many causes of anemia. Before treatment, the cause needs to be determined.

Drugs Used to Treat Anemia
ERYTHROPOIETIN
IRON
cyanocobalamin (vitamin B$_{12}$)
epoetin alfa, darbepoetin alfa
folic acid

Iron salts, such as ferrous sulfate, are used as iron supplements to treat iron deficiency anemia.

Folic acid and vitamin B$_{12}$ are used to treat anemias caused by deficiencies of these vitamins.

Erythropoietin is synthesized in the kidney in response to hypoxia or anemia. It then stimulates erythropoiesis (red cell proliferation).

Epoetin alfa and darbepoetin alfa are human recombinant erythropoietins.

Human erythropoietin is used in the treatment of anemia associated with end-stage renal failure.

DRUGS FOR SICKLE CELL DISEASE

Sickle cell disease is a group of inherited disorders caused by mutations in the beta globin gene, called hemoglobin S, that is expressed after birth.

Hydroxyurea will increase the expression of HbF in the treatment of sickle cell disease.

Hydroxyurea causes a shift in gene expression at the beta globin locus, resulting in increased production of fetal hemoglobin and decreased production of adult hemoglobin. Treatment with hydroxyurea improves erythrocyte morphology and deformability, reducing hemolysis.

Crizanlizumab (a monoclonal antibody) binds to P-selectin, a protein on the endothelial surface. Once crizanlizumab binds, it inhibits adhesion of other cells to the endothelium, reduces vaso-occulsion, and increases blood flow.

Voxelotor is orally active and prevents sickle hemoglobin from polymerizing by binding directly to HbS.

17 Lipid-Lowering Drugs

Organization of Class
Additional Explanation of Mechanisms

ORGANIZATION OF CLASS

Drugs used in the treatment of elevated serum lipids (hyperlipidemias) are targeted to decrease production of lipoprotein or cholesterol, increase degradation of a lipoprotein, or increase removal of cholesterol from the body.

The lipoproteins are large assemblies of lipids and proteins that bind and transport fats, such as lipids and triglycerides, in the blood. The lipids include free esterified cholesterol, triglycerides, and phospholipids. The proteins are known as *apolipoproteins* or *apoproteins*. They are classified according to lipid and protein content, transport function, and mechanism of lipid delivery. The high-density lipoproteins (HDL) are often referred to as the "good cholesterol" in contrast to the low- and very-low-density lipoproteins (LDL and VLDL), the "bad cholesterol." Now would be a good time to review the physiology and biochemistry of fats, lipoproteins, and lipoprotein receptors.

The most important facts about the relatively few drugs in this class are the mechanisms of action. Practically speaking, taste, dose, and cost are also important considerations.

Drugs	Mechanism
ATORVASTIN	Inhibit HMG-CoA reductase
cerivastatin	
fluvastatin	
lovastatin	
pitavastatin	
PRAVASTATIN	
ROSUVASTATIN	
SIMVASTATIN	

(Continued)

Drugs	Mechanism
CHOLESTYRAMINE	Bile acid–binding resins
colesevelam	
colestipol	
EZETIMIBE	Inhibits absorption of cholesterol
alirocumab	PCSK9 inhibitors
evolocumab	
niacin	?
fenofibrate	Activate nuclear transcription factor peroxisome proliferator-activated receptor-alpha (PPAR-alpha)
gemfibrozil	
bempedoic acid	ACL inhibitor

First, compare the list of drugs in the preceding box with that in your textbook or class handouts and add or delete drugs as needed. Next, compare the mechanisms of action noted here to those in your textbook or handouts. Some of these mechanisms are not entirely worked out so there may be discrepancies. Don't let that throw you off.

Basically, this box summarizes the most important things to know. If there is too much information here for you to absorb at one sitting, start by learning the two bile-binding resins and the drugs that inhibit HMG-CoA reductase (identified by their common ending of "-statin"). The rest of the drugs alter metabolism of lipoproteins. If you already have a good grasp of this content, you can skip the rest of this chapter.

ADDITIONAL EXPLANATION OF MECHANISMS

> The HMG-CoA reductase inhibitors are the first-choice drugs for the treatment of patients who require lipid-lowering therapy.

These drugs, referred to generally as "-statins," contain structural analogues of 3-hydroxy-3-methylglutarate (HMG), which is a precursor of cholesterol. They inhibit HMG-CoA reductase, the enzyme that controls the rate-limiting step in cholesterol synthesis. This depletes intracellular cholesterol. The cell then looks to the extracellular space for the cholesterol it needs. Since cholesterol is a required component of VLDLs, reduction in the synthesis of cholesterol by statins will also reduce hepatic VLDL production. Statins also improve endothelial function, decrease platelet aggregation, and reduce inflammation. The first side effect to know is myalgia, which is fairly common and can be precipitated by drug interactions.

The bile-binding resins (cholestyramine, colestipol, and colesevelam) are anion exchange resins that bind negatively charged bile acids in the small intestine.

The resins are not absorbed and are not metabolized. The resin-bile acid complex is excreted in the feces (Figure 17–1). The body compensates for the reduction in bile acids by converting cholesterol to bile acids, thus effectively lowering the cholesterol levels. Because of the mechanism of action, it should seem reasonable to you that these resins may also affect the absorption of other drugs and the fat-soluble vitamins.

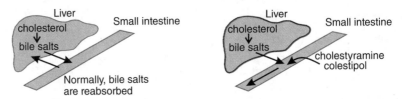

FIGURE 17–1 Normally, bile acids are secreted into the small intestine and then reabsorbed almost completely. Cholestyramine and colestipol bind to the bile acids in the small intestine and prevent their reabsorption. This causes the liver to use cholesterol to make more bile acids.

Ezetimibe inhibits the absorption of dietary and biliary cholesterol by blocking transport into the small intestine. This results in a compensatory increase in cholesterol synthesis that can be inhibited by statins.

Alirocumab and evolocumab are monoclonal antibodies (see the "mab" ending to their name?) that bind to proprotein convertase subtilisin/kexin type 9 (PCSK9). PCSK9 is a protease that binds to the LDL receptor and enhances degradation of the receptor resulting in higher plasma LDL concentrations. Loss of function of this protease is associated with reduced LDL levels and lower risk of atherosclerotic disease. These drugs are approved as an adjunct to diet and in addition to maximal doses of statins. As "mabs," these drugs have to be injected.

Niacin, a water-soluble B-complex vitamin, lowers both plasma cholesterol and triglyceride levels. The lipid-lowering effects are the result of decreased hepatic secretion of VLDL. This appears to be due to decreased triglyceride synthesis. Flushing is the most common side effect. Use of niacin in combination with statins may cause myopathy and (in the United States) the Food and Drug Administration (FDA) withdrew approval of niacin/statin combination formulations.

Gemfibrozil, fenofibrate, and clofibrate—the "-fibrates"—are used mainly to lower triglycerides and may increase HDL cholesterol. They activate the nuclear transcription factor peroxisome proliferator-activated receptor-alpha (a mouthful!!), also known as PPAR-alpha. PPAR-alpha regulates the genes that control lipid and glucose metabolism, inflammation, and endothelial function.

Bempedoic acid inhibits adenosine triphosphate citrate lyase (ACL), which is an enzyme involved in cholesterol synthesis in the liver. Bempedoic acid can be used alone or in combination with ezetimibe.

Long chain omega-3 polyunsaturated fatty acids can reduce elevated triglycerides and are available over the counter. These fish oil supplements are used in patients with severe hypertriglyceridemia. Icosapent ethyl is an approved prescription product to use as an adjunct to statin therapy.

If you have time and energy, mipomersen (subcutaneous [SC] injections) and lomitapide (oral) are approved solely for the treatment of homozygous familial hypercholesterolemia. This is a rare inherited condition that is most commonly caused by defects in the LDL receptor gene. Patients with this condition have very high LDL levels, cutaneous xanthoma, and (without treatment) early cardiovascular (CV) disease and death. Interestingly, mipomersen is an antisense oligonucleotide that inhibits synthesis of apo B-100. Both drugs can cause serious side effects, including hepatotoxicity. There is also a monoclonal antibody available for this condition. Evinacumab is the first ANGPTL3 (a protein that regulates lipid metabolism) inhibitor approved in the United States.

PART IV Drugs That Act on the Central Nervous System

CHAPTER 18:   Drugs Used in Dementia   97

CHAPTER 19:   Anxiolytic and Hypnotic Drugs   99

CHAPTER 20:   Drugs Used in Mood Disorders   106

CHAPTER 21:   Drugs Used in Thought Disorders   112

CHAPTER 22:   Drugs for Movement Disorders   116

CHAPTER 23:   Drugs for Seizure Disorders   121

CHAPTER 24:   Narcotics (Opiates)   125

CHAPTER 25:   General Anesthetics   129

CHAPTER 26:   Local Anesthetics   133

Drugs Used in Dementia

Organization of Class
Cholinesterase Inhibitors
NMDA Blocker

ORGANIZATION OF CLASS

Dementia, including Alzheimer disease, involves a number of brain systems. There is evidence for a decrease in markers of cholinergic neuron activity *and* for changes in brain glutamate, dopamine, norepinephrine, serotonin, and somatostatin. Eventually, cholinergic neurons die or are destroyed. Treatment has focused on increasing the amount of acetylcholine in the synapse by inhibiting the breakdown of acetylcholine.

> None of the drugs available for dementia alter the underlying pathology. They produce only a marginal improvement in symptoms.

Cholinesterase Inhibitors	NMDA Antagonist
DONEPEZIL	MEMANTINE
galantamine	
rivastigmine	
tacrine	

CHOLINESTERASE INHIBITORS

Acetylcholinesterase is the enzyme the breaks down synaptically released acetylcholine (see Chapter 7). Cholinesterase inhibitors have been used as nerve gases or in the treatment of myasthenia gravis. The group of cholinesterase inhibitors used in dementia appears to have selectivity for the brain enzyme and, therefore, have fewer systemic side effects than you would predict. The cholinesterase inhibitors are used in mild to moderate disease.

Of the drugs currently available, tacrine is the oldest but has limited use. Galantamine has some additional agonist activity at nicotinic receptors to enhance release of acetylcholine.

NMDA BLOCKER

Memantine is a noncompetitive antagonist at the *N*-methyl-D-aspartate (NMDA) sub-type of glutamate receptor.

The mechanism of action of memantine in dementia is not well understood. *N*-methyl-D-aspartate (NMDA) receptors are involved in learning and memory and blocking these receptors blocks memory formation. NMDA receptors also allow calcium influx into neurons and have been implicated in excitotoxicity in the presence of excess glutamate. Memantine is a low-affinity blocker of the channel, so it is thought that memantine can block excess calcium influx but can't block the physiologic actions of glutamate involved in learning.

Memantine appears to be effective in patients on cholinesterase inhibitors.

CHAPTER

19

Anxiolytic and Hypnotic Drugs

Tolerance and Dependence
Organization of Class
Barbiturates
Benzodiazepines
Buspirone
Drugs for Insomnia
    Benzodiazepine Receptor Agonists (Z Compounds)
    Melatonin Receptor Agonist
    Orexin Receptor Antagonist

TOLERANCE AND DEPENDENCE

Before we move on to the central nervous system (CNS) sedatives and narcotics, we need to clarify a few terms and definitions.

> Tolerance is a physiologic state characterized by a reduced drug effect with repeated use of the drug. Higher doses are needed to produce the same effect.

Essentially, tolerance is a state of reduced effectiveness. The term does not give any indication of the mechanism involved. Tolerance could be the result of increased elimination of a drug or of reduced effectiveness of drug-receptor interaction. For some drugs, tolerance develops to one effect of the drug and not to other effects. For example, with the narcotics, tolerance develops to the analgesic effect, but less tolerance develops to the respiratory depression.

> Cross-tolerance means that individuals tolerant to one drug will be tolerant to other drugs in the same class, but not to drugs in other classes.

A person who is tolerant to the sedative effects of one barbiturate will be tolerant to the effect of all the barbiturates (a situation termed cross-tolerance). However, that person will not be tolerant to the sedative effects of opiates.

> Dependence is characterized by signs and symptoms of withdrawal when drug levels fall.

Dependence can be physical or it can be psychological. There is something called cross-dependence, which is similar to cross-tolerance.

ORGANIZATION OF CLASS

Drugs that are classified as anxiolytics and hypnotics are used for a variety of purposes, including treatment of anxiety, epilepsy, sleep induction, and anesthesia. They are often called sedative-hypnotics or just anxiolytics. Looking at it the other way around, a variety of drug classes are used to treat anxiety, including benzodiazepines, serotonin-specific reuptake inhibitors (SSRI; see Chapter 20), serotonin/norepinephrine reuptake inhibitors (SNRI; see Chapter 20), β-blockers (see Chapter 10), and buspirone.

The anxiolytic and hypnotic drugs are generally classified by chemical structure. The two largest groups of drugs are the barbiturates and benzodiazepines. There are a relatively large number of drugs in both of these groups, but (thankfully) their names are generally recognizable. The barbiturates are no longer used to treat anxiety, but it is easier to learn them in this context.

Barbiturates	Benzodiazepines	Others	NBBRAs
PHENOBARBITAL	ALPRAZOLAM	BUSPIRONE	zaleplon
THIOPENTAL	DIAZEPAM	chloral hydrate	zolpidem
amobarbital	LORAZEPAM	ramelteon	eszopiclone
methohexital	clonazepam		
pentobarbital	clorazepate		
secobarbital	flurazepam		
	oxazepam		
	quazepam		
	temazepam		
	triazolam		

Notice that the barbiturates all end in "-tal" and all, *except* thiopental and methohexital, end in "-barbital." The benzodiazepines, for the most part, end in "-pam" or "-lam." The notable exception here is chlordiazepoxide. This nomenclature makes it easy to succeed at name recognition.

All of these drugs reduce anxiety at low doses and produce sedation at slightly higher doses (Figure 19–1). Most induce sleep (hypnosis), thus, the name sedative-hypnotics. At higher doses, the barbiturates produce some degree of anesthesia, and at even higher doses, produce medullary depression and death.

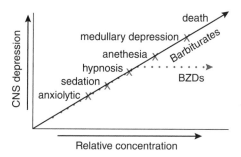

FIGURE 19–1 This graph schematizes the effects of benzodiazepines (BZDs) and barbiturates. Notice that the effects of the barbiturates continue up the line of CNS depression to death, whereas benzodiazepines veer off after hypnosis.

BARBITURATES

> Barbiturates enhance the function of γ-aminobutyric acid (GABA) in the CNS.

Barbiturates both enhance GABA responses and mimic GABA by opening the chloride channel in the absence of GABA. The net result of both actions is an increase in inhibition in the CNS.

> Barbiturates will
>   1. Produce sedation, hypnosis, coma, and *death*
>   2. Suppress respiration (overdose can lead to *death*)
>   3. Induce the liver P-450 system

All barbiturates suppress respiration by inhibiting the hypoxic and CO_2 response of the chemoreceptors. This means that a slight increase in the CO_2 content of the blood does not result in an increase in respirations when the patient has taken barbiturates.

> Any other drug that is metabolized by the P-450 system will be altered by the presence of barbiturates.

All barbiturates are metabolized by the liver and *all* induce the cytochrome P-450 microsomal enzymes. Thus, there is a long list of drug interactions for the barbiturates.

> The selection of a particular barbiturate depends on the duration of action of the agent, which in turn depends on its lipid solubility.

Barbiturates are classified according to their duration of action. Thiopental is an ultra-short-acting agent (minutes); pentobarbital, secobarbital, and amobarbital are short-acting agents (hours), and phenobarbital is a long-acting agent (days). Thiopental (ultra-short-acting) is highly lipid soluble. After administration, it rapidly enters the brain and then is redistributed into other body tissues and eventually into fat. As it is redistributed, the concentration in the brain drops below effective levels. Therefore, the duration of action of thiopental is very short.

Do not try to memorize the duration of action of the barbiturates. Learn the few that are clinically useful today. Thiopental and methohexital, the ultra-short-acting barbiturates, are used in anesthesia (see Chapter 25). The long-duration barbiturate phenobarbital is used to treat epilepsy (see Chapter 23).

> Symptoms of withdrawal in a person dependent on barbiturates include anxiety, nausea and vomiting, hypotension, seizures, and psychosis. Cardiovascular collapse may develop, leading to *death*.

Physical dependence on barbiturates develops with chronic use. The symptoms of barbiturate withdrawal can be quite serious and even *fatal*.

BENZODIAZEPINES

> Benzodiazepines bind to a specific site associated with the $GABA_A$ receptor, which results in increased inhibition.

Binding of benzodiazepines to this specific site enhances the affinity of GABA receptors for GABA, resulting in more frequent opening of the chloride channels. The increased influx of chloride causes hyperpolarization and increased inhibition.

All benzodiazepines reduce anxiety and produce sedation. In contrast to the barbiturates, the benzodiazepines reduce anxiety at doses that do not produce sedation. Some agents are used as antiepileptic agents, and some are used in the induction of anesthesia. Duration of action and pharmacokinetic properties are important considerations in selecting the drug to be used.

> Most benzodiazepines are metabolized in the liver to active metabolites. In general, the metabolites have slower elimination rates than the parent compound.

It is not necessary to memorize a metabolism scheme for the benzodiazepines. However, as a glance at Figure 19–2 will show, many of the agents in this class appear to be interrelated.

A few benzodiazepines are *not* extensively metabolized. They tend to have shorter half-lives.

This issue of elimination half-life for the benzodiazepines can be confusing. It may not always be clear whether a textbook is referring to the half-life of the parent compound only or the total half-life of the parent plus the active metabolites.

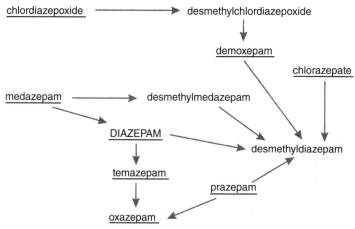

FIGURE 19–2 The metabolism and interrelationship of many of the benzodiazepines are shown in this figure. The compounds that are available pharmacologic preparations are underlined.

> Elimination half-life is not the same as duration of action for the benzodiazepines.

The elimination half-life is determined by the rate of liver metabolism or renal excretion, or both. In other words, the half-life measures the time that the drug is present in the body. It gives no indication about the time the drug is present at the GABA receptors in the brain, which represents the duration of action. A drug that is hidden in a fat pad may not be metabolized by the liver microsomal enzymes for several days. This drug would have a very long elimination half-life and a short duration of action because it has no action on the brain while hidden in fat.

> Physical and psychological dependence to benzodiazepines can occur.

Withdrawal from benzodiazepines can appear as confusion, anxiety, agitation, and restlessness. Benzodiazepines with short half-lives induce more abrupt and severe withdrawal reactions than do drugs with longer half-lives.

> FLUMAZENIL is a benzodiazepine antagonist.

Flumazenil can be used to reverse the sedative effects of benzodiazepines after anesthesia or after overdose with benzodiazepines.

It may be helpful to add some specific facts about the use of individual agents to the general knowledge we have reviewed so far.

> Some specific benzodiazepines have special uses. DIAZEPAM and LORAZEPAM are used in the treatment of status epilepticus. CHLORDIAZEPOXIDE is used in cases of alcohol withdrawal.

Over the years, different benzodiazepines have been preferred for the treatment of anxiety. Nowadays benzodiazepines are really only used for short-term treatment of acute anxiety.

BUSPIRONE

> BUSPIRONE is a nonbenzodiazepine that is used to treat generalized anxiety disorder.

Buspirone is relatively nonsedating and has few CNS side effects. Evidence suggests that buspirone primarily acts as a full agonist at presynaptic 5-HT receptors in the raphe nuclei and as a partial agonist at postsynaptic 5-HT1$_A$ receptors. It also has some activity at dopamine (D$_2$) receptors. Buspirone does not produce dependence. Because it does not act at the GABA receptor-chloride channel, buspirone is not recommended for the treatment of withdrawal from benzodiazepines.

It is interesting to compare benzodiazepines with buspirone. Benzodiazepines have an effect after a single dose and need days to achieve a full therapeutic effect, whereas buspirone does not have an effect with a single dose and needs weeks to achieve a full therapeutic effect.

DRUGS FOR INSOMNIA

Pharmacologic treatment of insomnia includes a variety of prescription and nonprescription drugs, "natural" remedies and behavioral therapy. Some drugs are used off-label for their sedative effects. For example, the antipsychotic quetiapine has been used for its sedative "side-effect." The tricyclic antidepressant doxepin is Food and Drug Administration (FDA) approved for the treatment of sleep maintenance insomnia. Antihistamines, particularly first-generation ones, have sedation as a significant side effect and they can be used as a sleep aide. Several herbal products are reported to have mild hypnotic effects, including valerian root, L-tryptophan, chamomile tea, and skull cap.

BENZODIAZEPINE RECEPTOR AGONISTS (Z COMPOUNDS)

Normally it's great when a class of drugs is named according to the mechanism of action, but in this case it's mouthful. Zaleplon, zolpidem, and eszopiclone are known as nonbenzodiazepine benzodiazepine receptor agonists (NBBRAs). In other words, they are not structurally related to benzodiazepines (Figure 19–3), but they are agonists at the benzodiazepine receptor. All three drugs will shorten the time it takes to fall asleep. These drugs are used for short-term treatment of insomnia.

MELATONIN RECEPTOR AGONIST

Melatonin, synthesized in the pineal gland, acts on MT$_1$ and MT$_2$ receptors in the hypothalamus to affect both sleep and circadian rhythms. The MT$_1$ receptor

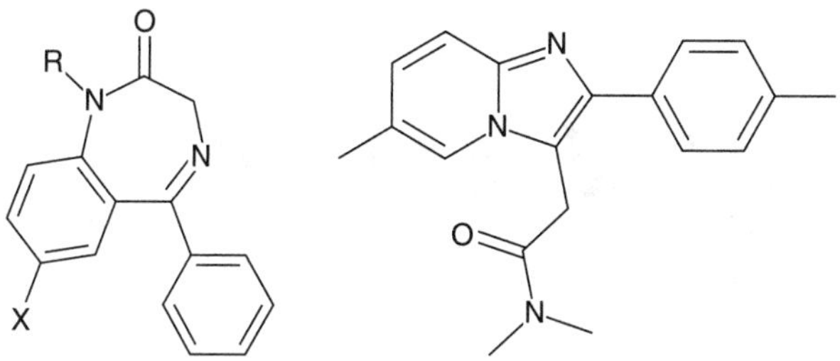

benzodiazepine zolpidem

FIGURE 19-3 On the left is the general structure of a benzodiazepine. On the right is a nonbenzodiazepine benzodiazepine agonist—zolpidem. As you can see, the structures are quite different.

appears to be more important for sleep regulation, while the MT_2 receptor may mediate circadian rhythms. Ramelteon and tasimelteon bind to both MT_1 and MT_2 and are used for insomnia.

OREXIN RECEPTOR ANTAGONIST

Orexin peptides sustain wakefulness, so blocking the orexin receptor will promote sleep. Suvorexant and lemborexant are antagonists at both orexin 1 and 2 receptors. Patients treated with suvorexant fall asleep 5 to 10 minutes sooner and stay asleep 15 to 25 minutes longer. Interestingly, loss of orexin signaling has been associated with narcolepsy.

20 Drugs Used in Mood Disorders

Organization of Antidepressants

Serotonin-Specific Reuptake Inhibitors

Serotonin/Norepinephrine Reuptake Inhibitors (SNRI)

Heterocyclics/TCAs

Monoamine Oxidase Inhibitors

Other Antidepressants

Drugs Used in Bipolar Disorder

ORGANIZATION OF ANTIDEPRESSANTS

All of the antidepressant drugs increase the concentration of norepinephrine or serotonin in the synaptic cleft. In most cases, they do this by inhibiting the reuptake of the neurotransmitters. Remember that reuptake is the major route for termination of action of these neurotransmitters. Other drugs block their metabolic degradation or increase their release.

It is most logical to divide the antidepressants into five, or more, groups. Three groups are named according to their mechanism of action. Therefore, if you can remember the name of the group, you have already learned an important fact about each drug in the group. One group, the heterocyclics, consists mostly of tricyclic compounds (tricyclic antidepressants [TCA]). They are grouped together mainly on the basis of structure, but they also have similar actions and side effects.

The trouble most students seem to have with these drugs is with their names. As you can see from the following table, the names of these drugs give no clues to their class. This is one instance where name recognition becomes very important for examination preparation. You may know everything about the serotonin/ norepinephrine reuptake inhibitors (SNRIs), but if you do not recognize that venlafaxine belongs to that group, you may not be able to answer a question about this drug.

SSRIs	SNRIs	Heterocyclics	MAO Inhibitors	Others
FLUOXETINE	desvenlafaxine	DESIPRAMINE	isocarboxazid	BUPROPION
citalopram	duloxetine	IMIPRAMINE	phenelzine	mirtazapine
escitalopram	levomilnacipran	amitriptyline	tranylcypromine	nefazodone
paroxetine	milnacipran	nortriptyline		trazodone
sertraline	venlafaxine			vilazodone
				vortioxetine
				esketamine

Learn what you can about each class of antidepressant and then be sure that you know the names of the drugs in each class.

SEROTONIN-SPECIFIC REUPTAKE INHIBITORS

> Serotonin-specific reuptake inhibitors (SSRIs) are antidepressants that block the reuptake of serotonin.

These drugs block the reuptake of serotonin, without affecting reuptake of norepinephrine or dopamine. Therefore, they are referred to as *serotonin-specific reuptake inhibitors* or *selective serotonin reuptake inhibitors*. Either name gives you the abbreviation SSRI. It is currently believed that the mechanism by which these drugs alleviate depression is by their blockade of the reuptake of serotonin. This may seem self-evident. It takes several weeks of treatment with SSRIs to achieve a full therapeutic effect, and there is no evidence that one SSRI is more effective than any other.

The initial treatment of choice for most patients with depression is an SSRI. Drugs in this class are effective in a wide range of disorders in addition to depression. They are anxiolytic with efficacy in generalized anxiety disorder, panic disorder, social anxiety, and obsessive-compulsive disorder. SSRIs also have efficacy in eating disorders and borderline personality disorder.

> SSRIs are not cholinergic antagonists or α-blockers.

SSRIs are essentially devoid of agonist or antagonist activity at any neurotransmitter receptor. Sexual dysfunction is a side effect of the drugs in this class. Severe withdrawal symptoms can occur if the SSRI is stopped abruptly.

SEROTONIN/NOREPINEPHRINE REUPTAKE INHIBITORS (SNRI)

> Venlafaxine is an effective antidepressant that blocks reuptake of both serotonin and norepinephrine.

The serotonin/norepinephrine reuptake inhibitors (SNRIs) block reuptake of both serotonin and norepinephrine, hence the name of the class. Desvenlafaxine is an active metabolite of venlafaxine, but with no clinical advantage over the parent compound. The side effects with SNRIs are reported to be similar to those with SSRIs. SNRIs can cause a dose-dependent increase in blood pressure, presumably due to blocking reuptake of norepinephrine. Levomilnacipran is the active enantiomer from the racemic mixture called milnacipran, which is used for fibromyalgia. Other off-label uses for the SNRIs include stress urinary incontinence (duloxetine), autisn, binge-eating disorders, diabetic neuropathy (duloxetine), fibromyalgia (duloxetine), hot flashes, pain syndromes, premenstrual dysphoric disorders, and posttraumatic stress disorder (PTSD) (venlafaxine).

> A related drug, atomoxetine, which is a selective/norepinephrine reuptake inhibitor (SNRIs), is used to treat attention-deficit/hyperactivity disorder (ADHD).

HETEROCYCLICS/TCAs

> The precise mechanism of action of the tricyclic drugs is unknown. These drugs block the reuptake of biogenic amines, including norepinephrine and serotonin.

Most of the drugs in this class are really tricyclics, based on their chemical structure of a three-ring core (Figure 20–1). A couple of other useful antidepressants do not have the three-ring core but otherwise are similar in action and side effects to

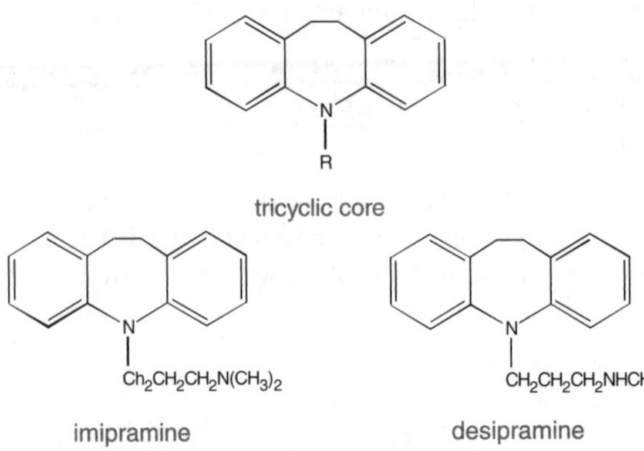

tricyclic core

imipramine   desipramine

FIGURE 20–1 The main structure of the tricyclic antidepressants and two examples of drugs in this class. The three rings are obvious.

the tricyclic compounds. Therefore, they should all be learned together. The drugs are equally efficacious but vary in potency. In addition, some patients will respond to one drug in this class and not to another one.

Tricyclics have little effect in normal (nondepressed) people. As with most of the antidepressants, 2 to 3 weeks of dosing with the tricyclics are required before an effect on depression is detectable.

> Heterocyclic antidepressants are
>
>   1. Potent muscarinic cholinergic antagonists
>   2. Weak α_1 antagonists
>   3. Weak H_1 antagonists
>
> These actions account for the major side effects of these drugs.

If you can remember these three actions of the heterocyclic antidepressants, you can also list most of the significant side effects based on your knowledge of autonomic pharmacology (see Chapter 8). The cholinergic blocking effect produces dry mouth, constipation, urinary retention, blurred vision, and so on. The α-blocking effect produces orthostatic hypotension, and the H_1-antagonism produces sedation. Tolerance to the anticholinergic effects does occur.

In overdose, these drugs can produce serious, life-threatening cardiac arrhythmias, delirium, and psychosis. As a group they have a very narrow therapeutic index (see Chapter 2), which means that safety is an issue.

MONOAMINE OXIDASE INHIBITORS

> Monoamine oxidase (MAO) inhibitors increase levels of norepinephrine, serotonin, and dopamine by inhibiting their degradation.

Although rarely used anymore, MAO inhibitors are antidepressants.

Monoamine oxidase is a mitochondrial enzyme that exists in two major forms: A and B. Its major role is to oxidize monoamines, including norepinephrine, serotonin, and dopamine. Blocking this degradative enzyme slows the removal of these transmitters.

Isocarboxazid, phenelzine, and tranylcypromine are irreversible, nonselective inhibitors of MAO-A and MAO-B. However, research suggests that the antidepressant effect of these drugs is due to inhibition of MAO-A.

> MAO inhibitors can cause a *fatal* hypertensive crisis.

Patients who take MAO inhibitors should not take SSRIs or eat foods rich in tyramine or other biologically active amines. These foods include cheese, beer, and red wine. Normally tyramine and other amines are rapidly inactivated by MAO in the gut. Individuals who are taking MAO inhibitors are unable to inactivate the tyramine. The tyramine causes release of norepinephrine, which can lead to an increase in blood pressure and cardiac arrhythmias.

OTHER ANTIDEPRESSANTS

A number of agents are available now, each in its own unique class. Here we will lump them together as other antidepressants.

> Bupropion is an effective antidepressant that is also approved for use (in combination with behavioral modification) in smoking-cessation programs.

Bupropion is structurally unrelated to the other antidepressants. It is sometimes classified as a norepinephrine-dopamine reuptake inhibitor, but it's hard to have a class with only 1 drug. Bupropion has very few side effects; in particular, it causes less sexual dysfunction than the SSRIs. There is an increased risk of seizures with higher-than-recommended doses. As with the other antidepressants, the therapeutic effect takes several weeks. Bupropion can also be used to treat nicotine withdrawal.

Nefazodone, trazodone, and mirtazapine are classed as serotonin receptor antagonists (5-HT$_2$) and reuptake inhibitors. They are structurally unrelated to SSRIs, heterocyclics, or MAO inhibitors. Trazodone is sedative, but nefazodone less so. Nefazodone inhibits serotonin and norepinephrine reuptake and antagonizes 5-HT$_2$ and α_1 receptors. The α_1-antagonism should tell you that this drug may cause orthostatic hypotension. As with the other antidepressants, the therapeutic effect takes several weeks.

> Trazodone – priapism (rarely)
>
> Nefazodone – black box warning for hepatotoxicity
>
> Mirtazapine – sleepiness, increased appetite, and weight gain

Low doses of trazodone can be used for insomnia. Its efficacy in elderly patients is well documented, and it can be used for anxiety disorders.

Esketamine is the newest antidepressant, approved in 2019, with a novel mechanism of action. It is an enantiomer of ketamine, a noncompetitive NMDA antagonist and drug of abuse. It was approved for use as a nasal spray for use in combination with an oral antidepressant drug in patients with treatment resistant depression.

> Sibutramine is a norepinephrine, 5-HT, and dopamine reuptake inhibitor that is used as a weight-loss agent.

Although sibutramine is not an antidepressant, it is included here because of the similarity of its mechanism of action. Sibutramine has its effects on the central nervous system, where it inhibits the reuptake of neurotransmitters. The inhibition of reuptake of 5-HT is thought to enhance satiety; the inhibition of reuptake of norepinephrine is thought to increase metabolic rate.

DRUGS USED IN BIPOLAR DISORDER

The main goal of pharmacological treatment of bipolar disorder is to reduce the frequency and severity of fluctuations in mood.

> LITHIUM, carbamazepine, valproate and lamotrigine are drugs used for the treatment of bipolar disorder.

Lithium is still considered the standard treatment for bipolar disorder. However, the anticonvulsants, carbamazepine, valproate, and lamotrigine are also used (see Chapter 23). How any of these drugs work to reduce mood changes is not known. Second-generation antipsychotic drugs (see Chapter 21) are also used for treatment of acute mania and for maintenance treatment of bipolar disorder.

> LITHIUM has a low therapeutic index, and the frequency and severity of adverse reactions are directly related to the serum levels.

Frequent measurements of the serum level are routinely carried out during chronic treatment. Lithium use is commonly associated with polyuria and polydipsia and rarely with hypothyroidism or nephrogenic diabetes insipidus.

C H A P T E R

21

Drugs Used in Thought Disorders

Organization of Class
Typical Antipsychotics (First Generation)
Serotonin-Dopamine Antagonists (Second Generation)
Neuroleptic Malignant Syndrome

ORGANIZATION OF CLASS

These drugs have been called neuroleptics, antischizophrenic drugs, antipsychotic drugs, and major tranquilizers. All these terms are synonymous; neuroleptic and antipsychotic are the most common. These drugs are not curative (because they do not eliminate the fundamental thinking disorder), but they often permit the patient to function more normally.

All of the neuroleptics are

1. α-Blockers
2. Muscarinic antagonists
3. Histamine antagonists

These actions produce the side effects of the drugs.

If you know which receptors these drugs block, you can predict all of the actions and side effects of these drugs. The antimuscarinic actions produce dry mouth, constipation, urinary retention, blurred vision, and so on. The α-antagonism produces orthostatic hypotension, and the H_1-antagonism produces sedation.

These drugs were organized according to their chemical structure. I do not recommend this method unless you have decided to memorize all of the structures. I recommend dividing these drugs into two groups: the older, so-called typical antipsychotics and the newer atypical drugs. The newer "atypical" drugs are now the drugs of choice for the treatment of schizophrenia, so the term "atypical" is a misnomer. The older drugs are also called "first generation" and the newer drugs "second generation." This makes much more sense. Name recognition here is sometimes a problem but notice that most of the typical neuroleptics end in "-azine." A number of the second-generation drugs end in "–peridone."

All neuroleptics are dopamine blockers (D_2), but the atypical drugs (second generation) also block 5-HT_{2A} receptors.

Typical Neuroleptics (First Generation)	5-HT-DA Antagonists (Second Generation)
acetophenazine	aripiprazole
CHLORPROMAZINE	asenapine
chlorprothixene	brexpiprazole
fluphenazine	CLOZAPINE
HALOPERIDOL	iloperidone
mesoridazine	lurasidone
perphenazine	olanzapine
prochlorperazine	paliperidone
thioridazine	quetiapine
thiothixene	RISPERIDONE
trifluoperazine	ziprasidone

You now know the most fundamental information about the drugs in this group. You need only add a little bit more, depending on how much trivia you want to know.

TYPICAL ANTIPSYCHOTICS (FIRST GENERATION)

All the drugs in this group have equal efficacy; they vary only in potency and side effects.

REMINDER: The typical antipsychotics block dopamine, muscarinic cholinergic, α-adrenergic, and H_1-histaminergic receptors.

The dopamine antagonism is believed to produce the antipsychotic effect. It also produces some endocrine effects. Remember that dopamine inhibits prolactin release. Thus, an antagonist at the dopamine receptor results in an increase in prolactin release. This in turn leads to lactation. Most of the neuroleptics, *except* thioridazine, have antiemetic effects that are mediated by blocking D_2 receptors of the chemoreceptor trigger zone in the medulla.

All of these drugs produce extrapyramidal effects, including parkinsonism, akathisia, and tardive dyskinesia.

The extrapyramidal effects of these drugs are presumably caused by blocking of dopamine receptors in the striatum (basal ganglia). Extrapyramidal effects include acute dystonia (spasm of the muscles of the face, tongue, neck, and back), akathisia (motor restlessness), and parkinsonism (rigidity, tremor, and shuffling gait). Because it is irreversible, one of the most worrisome extrapyramidal effects is tardive dyskinesia. Tardive dyskinesia may appear during or after prolonged therapy with any of these drugs. It involves stereotyped involuntary movements, such as lip smacking, jaw movements, and darting of the tongue. Purposeless quick movements of the limbs may also occur.

> In 2017, valbenazine and deutetrabenazine, VMAT2 inhibitors, were approved for the treatment of tardive dyskinesia. Another VMAT2 inhibitor, tetrabenazine is used to treat chorea in Huntington disease.

In case you do not remember, VMAT2 is a protein found in the brain that is responsible for uptake of monoamine neurotransmitters into vesicles in presynaptic neurons. Inhibition of VMAT2 keeps the neurotransmitters in the synaptic cleft longer.

The more potent drugs produce more extrapyramidal effects. Conversely, the drugs with more anticholinergic potency have fewer extrapyramidal effects. Compare this to what we know about Parkinson disease (see Chapter 22). In Parkinson disease, a loss of dopamine neurons leads to a movement disorder that can be treated with anticholinergics. Here, we are using drugs to block dopamine receptors, which you may predict will lead to parkinsonism (symptoms that are similar to Parkinson disease, but not caused by a loss of neurons). Drugs with anticholinergic actions cause fewer extrapyramidal effects because the dopamine-acetylcholine balance in the motor systems is less affected.

SEROTONIN-DOPAMINE ANTAGONISTS (SECOND GENERATION)

> Second-generation neuroleptics reduce both the positive and negative symptoms of schizophrenia, while causing a minimum of extrapyramidal side effects.

Although referred to as a serotonin-dopamine antagonist, each agent in this class has a unique combination of receptor affinities. At the very least you should know that these drugs are antagonists at dopamine and $5\text{-}HT_{2A}$ receptors. The affinities for the other receptors determine the side-effect profile. This is the type of information that you can add later. The ability of these drugs to reduce the negative features of psychosis (withdrawal, flat affect, anhedonia, catatonia) and the positive symptoms (hallucinations, delusions, disordered thought, agitation) has led to the use of these drugs in a wide variety of patients.

Clozapine has caused *fatal* agranulocytosis. In patients receiving clozapine, monitoring of the white cell count needs to be done on a regular basis. Agranulocytosis does not appear to be a problem with the newer agents in this class.

> **REMINDER:** The second-generation antipsychotics also block muscarinic, α_1-adrenergic, serotonin, and histamine receptors in addition to dopamine and serotonin receptors.

The side effects you learned for the whole class apply to these drugs as well.

> RISPERIDONE is the drug of choice for new onset schizophrenia.

In general, the second generation drugs have a lower risk of extrapyramidal symptoms and for tardive dyskinesia, but a higher risk of metabolic changes.

NEUROLEPTIC MALIGNANT SYNDROME

> Neuroleptic malignant syndrome is a rare, potentially *fatal* neurologic side effect of antipsychotic medication.

Many courses do not cover neuroleptic malignant syndrome, but because it is potentially fatal, it is worth a mention here. Neuroleptic malignant syndrome resembles a very severe form of parkinsonism, with catatonia, autonomic instability, and stupor. It may persist for more than a week after administration of the offending drug is stopped. Because mortality is high (10%-20%), immediate medical attention is required. This syndrome has occurred with all neuroleptics but is more common with relatively high doses of the more potent agents, especially when administered parenterally.

CHAPTER

22 Drugs for Movement Disorders

Therapy for Parkinson Disease
    Dopamine Replacement Therapy
    Dopamine Agonist Therapy
    Anticholinergic Therapy
Therapy for ALS and MS
Therapy for Duchenne Muscular Dystrophy and Spinal Muscular Atrophy

THERAPY FOR PARKINSON DISEASE

In Parkinson disease there is loss of the dopamine-containing neurons in the substantia nigra (Figure 22–1). These neurons normally project to the caudate putamen (one piece of the basal ganglia) where the dopamine inhibits firing of the cholinergic neurons. These cholinergic neurons form excitatory synapses onto other neurons that project out of the basal ganglia. The result of the loss

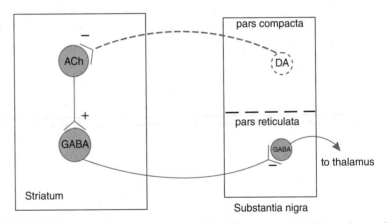

FIGURE 22–1 Diagram of projections into and out of the striatum. In Parkinson disease, there is a loss of the dopamine (DA)-containing neurons that project from the substantia nigra to the striatum where they inhibit cholinergic (ACh) neurons (*dashed line*).

of dopamine-containing neurons is that the cholinergic neurons are now without their normal inhibition. This is a bit like a car going down a hill without any brakes.

> **THERAPY FOR PARKINSON DISEASE**
> 1. Dopamine replacement therapy
> 2. Dopamine agonist therapy
> 3. Anticholinergic therapy

The goals of therapy are to correct the imbalance of the cholinergic neurons in the striatum. All of the therapeutic approaches to Parkinson disease make sense. Given the loss of dopamine-containing neurons, you could replace the dopamine or give dopamine agonists (to mimic the action of the lost dopamine). Because many of the cholinergic neurons are uninhibited, you could give an anticholinergic drug to try to restore inhibition. If you can remember this much, you are well on your way to a good grasp of this area.

DOPAMINE REPLACEMENT THERAPY

It would be nice if we could just give dopamine itself. However, dopamine does not cross the blood-brain barrier.

> LEVODOPA (L-dopa) is a metabolic precursor of dopamine that crosses the blood–brain barrier (Figure 22–2).

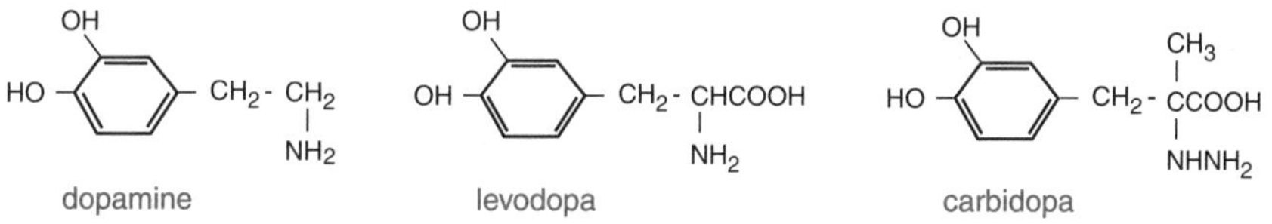

FIGURE 22–2 Structures of dopamine, levodopa, and carbidopa.

Large doses of levodopa are required because much of the drug is decarboxylated to dopamine in the periphery. All this dopamine floating around peripherally causes side effects.

> CARBIDOPA is a dopamine decarboxylase inhibitor that does not cross the blood–brain barrier. It reduces the peripheral metabolism of levodopa, thereby increasing the amount of levodopa that reaches the brain.

Carbidopa and levodopa are used today in combination. This is a prime example of a beneficial drug interaction that is logical based on the mechanisms of action of the two drugs. Side effects of levodopa and carbidopa are related to the dopamine that is generated by peripheral decarboxylation.

Tolcapone, entacapone, and opicapone are plasma catechol-O-methyltransferase (COMT) inhibitors that prolong the half-life of levodopa. Much lower on the trivia list is a new drug approved in 2020—istradefylline. Istradefylline is an oral adenosine A2A receptor antagonist for use as an adjunct in patients with "off" episodes.

> SELEGILINE is an inhibitor of monoamine oxidase (MAO)-B, the enzyme that metabolizes dopamine in the central nervous system (CNS).

Selegiline is also known as deprenyl, and both names appear in books and articles in the medical literature. Inhibition of MAO-B slows the breakdown of dopamine; thus, dopamine remains in the vicinity of its receptors on the cholinergic neurons for longer. Selegiline and rasagiline are irreversible MAO-B inhibitors for Parkinson disease, while safinamide is a reversible inhibitor to be used as an adjunct to carbidopa/levodopa.

Amantadine is an antiviral drug effective in the treatment of influenza. It appears to enhance the synthesis, release, or reuptake of dopamine from the surviving nigral neurons, so it can also be used in Parkinson disease.

DOPAMINE AGONIST THERAPY

Dopamine agonists can be used in Parkinson disease because although the dopamine-releasing neurons have disappeared, the postsynaptic dopamine receptors are still present and functional. Administration of dopamine agonists to stimulate these receptors should therefore restore the balance of inhibition and excitation in the basal ganglia.

The main role of these drugs is in combination with levodopa and carbidopa in early Parkinson disease. Dopamine agonists used in the treatment of Parkinson disease include bromocriptine, pramipexole, ropinirole, and rotigotine. The actions and side effects of these drugs are similar to those of levodopa. Remember that activation of dopamine receptors in the pituitary gland inhibits prolactin release. This reduction in prolactin can alter reproductive function.

ANTICHOLINERGIC THERAPY

Anticholinergic agents are less commonly used than the drugs previously reviewed, but they are always taught in pharmacology courses. They reduce the activity of the uninhibited cholinergic neurons in the basal ganglia. These drugs are muscarinic antagonists and differ only in potency. You should be able to list the side effects of muscarinic antagonists from your study of autonomic pharmacology (see Chapter 8). Therefore, there is little that is new here. However, the drug names are quite awkward and not easily recognizable as antimuscarinic agents.

> Trihexyphenidyl, benztropine, and biperiden are muscarinic antagonists used in Parkinson disease.

Side effects of these drugs include dry mouth, constipation, urinary retention, and confusion. The dopamine agonists and anticholinergics are good candidates for your drug name recognition list.

THERAPY FOR ALS AND MS

Amyotrophic lateral sclerosis (ALS, Lou Gehrig disease) is a disorder of upper and lower motor neurons, characterized by rapidly progressive weakness, muscle atrophy, spasticity, dysarthria, dysphagia, and respiratory difficulties. The spasticity can be treated with baclofen ($GABA_B$ agonist), tizanidine (α_2 agonist in central nervous system [CNS]) or a benzodiazepine such as clonazepam.

> Riluzole is an orally active agent that extends survival in ALS by 2 to 3 months.

Riluzole has complex actions in the CNS, including inhibition of glutamate release, blocking *N*-methyl-D-aspartate (NMDA) and kainate (KA) receptors and inhibition of voltage-gated sodium channels.

> Ocrelizumab and ofatumumab, anti-CD20 B-cell antibodies, are first-line therapy for multiple sclerosis.

Multiple sclerosis is an inflammatory disease characterized by demyelination and axonal loss. So far, the most effective treatment is with antibodies to CD20/CD52/integrin α_4. Immunomodulators, such as interferon and glatiramer acetate, are also used. Treatment options here are (relatively) rapidly changing, so check your text or online for the latest. Three oral sphingosine 1-phosphate (S1P) modulators have been approved for the treatment of the relapsing form of multiple sclerosis. They are more convenient (oral), but less effective that the "-mabs" (injection). If you can, learn to recognize the names—fingolimod, siponimod, and teriflunomide.

THERAPY FOR DUCHENNE MUSCULAR DYSTROPHY AND SPINAL MUSCULAR ATROPHY

Duchenne muscular dystrophy is a progressive X-linked recessive neuromuscular disorder characterized by decreased or absent levels of dystrophin. New treatment has appeared in the form of antisense oligonucleotides, golodirsen and viltolarsen, for patients with specific mutations in the dystrophin gene. This allows for production of a truncated dystrophin protein.

Spinal muscular atrophy is an autosomal recessive disorder characterized by muscle weakness and atrophy. Severity of the disease is related to the number of copies of functional gene. Nusinersen is an antisense oligonucleotide that increases production of SMN protein. More recently treatment with onasemnogene abeparvovec-xioi was approved. Onasemnogene abeparvovec is an adeno-associated virus vector-based gene therapy for one-time treatment of children younger than 2 years. You have probably heard about it because of the cost—a single dose costs $2,125,000.

Drugs for Seizure Disorders

Organization of Class
Important Details about the Most Important Drugs
Other Drugs to Consider

ORGANIZATION OF CLASS

This class of drugs, often called anticonvulsants, does not lend itself to the type of organization used in many other chapters. Here we need to consider the disease to be treated.

Epilepsy is a chronic disorder characterized by recurrent episodes in which the brain is subject to abnormal excessive discharges (seizures) synchronized throughout a population of neurons. The seizures themselves have been classified to assist with demographics and treatment. The accompanying table provides a simplified seizure classification scheme.

Seizure Type	Clinical Manifestations
I. Partial (focal, local)	
A. Partial simple	Focal motor, sensory, or speech disturbance. No impairment of consciousness.
B. Partial complex	
C. Partial seizures with secondary generalization	Dreamy state with automatisms. Impaired consciousness.
II. Generalized seizures	
A. Generalized convulsive (tonic-clonic, grand mal)	Loss of consciousness, falling, rigid extension of trunk and limbs. Rhythmic contractions of arms and legs.
B. Generalized nonconvulsive (absence, petit mal)	Impaired consciousness with staring and eye blinks.

Notice that some of these seizures do not involve muscle jerking or convulsions. In particular, absence seizures are called nonconvulsive. Technically, this would make the name *anticonvulsants* inaccurate, but it is often used to designate this class of drugs.

Now that we have defined the types of seizures we want to control, we can start examining the drugs. To simplify this organization, let's consider which drugs are used for which types of seizures. There is not 100% agreement on which is the best drug in each category, so do not be bothered by discrepancies between textbooks.

Focal Seizures	Conventional Drugs	More Recent Drugs
Simple focal	**carbamazepine**	brivaracetam
Complex focal	**phenytoin**	eslicarbazepine
	valproate	gabapentin
Focal with second generalization	**carbamazepine**	lacosamide
	phenobarbital	lamotrigine
	phenytoin	levetiracetam
	primidone	perampanel
	valproate	rufinamide
		tiagabine
		topiramate
		zonisamide
Generalized Seizures		
Absence	**ethosuximide**	lamotrigine
	valproate	
	clonazepam	
Myoclonic	**valproate**	levetiracetam
	clonazepam	
Tonic-clonic	**carbamazepine**	lamotrigine
	phenobarbital	levetiracetam
	phenytoin	topiramate
	primidone	
	valproate	

First, notice all the overlap; that is, drugs are used for more than one seizure type. Valproate is used for all types of seizures, and lamotrigine is used for all except one (check which one!).

IMPORTANT DETAILS ABOUT THE MOST IMPORTANT DRUGS

VALPROATE is associated with elevated liver enzymes, nausea and vomiting, and weight gain. It can also produce a tremor.

Valproate may produce *fatal* hepatic failure. This is most common in children under the age of 2 years who are taking more than one antiepileptic drug. The hepatotoxicity is not dose related; it is considered to be an idiosyncratic reaction. Valproate is also teratogenic, producing neural tube defects.

> CARBAMAZEPINE causes autoinduction of its own metabolism.

Carbamazepine is metabolized by the liver and over a period of several weeks induces the enzymes that metabolize it. Therefore, an initially adequate dose gradually produces lower and lower plasma levels as the liver increases the metabolism (shortening the half-life). Carbamazepine has been associated with granulocyte suppression and aplastic anemia. Besides seizures, carbamazepine has been used for bipolar disorder and trigeminal neuralgia.

Oxcarbazepine is chemically similar to carbamazepine but does not induce liver enzymes to the same extent.

> ETHOSUXIMIDE is the *drug of choice* for absence seizures. It is associated with stomach-aches, vomiting, and hiccups.

Ethosuximide is thought to act by blocking calcium channels in the thalamus.

Lamotrigine is a well-tolerated antiepileptic agent that is as effective as carbamazepine. It has also been reported to improve depression in some patients with epilepsy.

Levetiracetam binds to a synaptic vesicle protein called SV2A, but the relevance of this for its anticonvulsant activity is not yet known.

OTHER DRUGS TO CONSIDER

Phenytoin used to be widely used in the treatment of epilepsy but has been largely replaced in the United States with the newer drugs. However, much is known about the pharmacology of phenytoin, particularly the pharmacokinetics.

> PHENYTOIN has zero-order kinetics.

Review the section on zero-order kinetics in Chapter 4 if you need to. The fact that phenytoin has zero-order kinetics is particularly important because phenytoin turns into a zero-order drug right in the therapeutic range (Figure 23–1).

Phenytoin is thought to act by blocking the sodium channel in the inactivated state. If you are interested, you can learn additional details about its side effects and actions.

We are getting lower down on the trivia list. If you have learned most of the material we have reviewed so far, please continue. If you have had any trouble with the preceding material, you may wish to wait and add the following details during your second or third pass through.

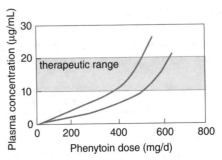

FIGURE 23-1 Plasma concentrations at steady state as a function of dose are shown for two different people. Notice that as the dose of phenytoin increases, the plasma concentration does not follow in a linear fashion. Instead, the curve becomes steeper where phenytoin is switching to zero-order kinetics. This transition occurs at different points for different people.

> PHENYTOIN causes ataxia and nystagmus at high doses. It has been associated with hirsutism, coarsening of facial features, and gingival hyperplasia.

There are several relatively new drugs that are effective antiepileptic agents in some patients. These include brivaracetam (analogue of levetiracetam), eslicarbazepine, felbamate (has caused aplastic anemia), gabapentin (also used for pain control), fosphenytoin (soluble prodrug for phenytoin), lacosamide, perampanel, topiramate, tiagabine, and zonisamide.

> Clonazepam is an alternative drug for the treatment of generalized nonconvulsive seizures. It is a benzodiazepine and tolerance develops to its antiepileptic effects.

Chapter 19, on anxiolytics and hypnotics, contains additional features about the benzodiazepines. Use what you learned there and apply it here. Again, do not memorize this drug in isolation. In Chapter 11 on diuretics, acetazolamide was mentioned. It can also be used for the treatment of seizures (and mountain sickness and glaucoma).

You should also take a few minutes to review the drugs used in the treatment of status epilepticus before moving on. Status epilepticus is when seizure recurs so close together that baseline consciousness is not regained between seizures. The seizures need to be treated intravenously (IV).

Narcotics (Opiates)

Organization of Class
Actions of Morphine and the Other Agonists
Distinguishing Features of Some Agonists
Opioid Antagonists
Opioid Agonist-Antagonists

ORGANIZATION OF CLASS

The word *narcotics* (or *opiates*) refers to drugs that act on specific receptors in the central nervous system (CNS) to reduce perception of pain. In general, they do not eliminate pain, but the patient is not as bothered by the pain. They act on three major classes of receptors in the CNS, called opioid receptors and designated mu (μ), kappa (κ), and delta (δ). Most of the actions of the narcotic analgesics are mediated by the μ receptor. Some actions are mediated through the κ and δ receptors.

Divide the narcotics into four groups:
1. Agonists; use morphine as the prototype
2. Weak agonist/reuptake inhibitors
3. Mixed agonist-antagonists
4. Antagonists

The most important drug names in this class are in capital letters in the following table. Notice that there are many more agonists than antagonists and that there is only one important mixed agonist-antagonist.

Remember the names of the antagonists (NALOXONE and NALTREXONE) and the most important mixed agonist-antagonist (PENTAZOCINE). Everything else is an agonist.

Of course, that statement was somewhat simplified. Use morphine as the prototype drug in this class. The other agonists have the same general properties. They vary in things like potency and duration of action.

The following table presents a partial listing of opiates.

Agonists	Weak Agonists/ Reuptake Inhibitors	Mixed Agonist-Antagonists	Antagonists
alfentanil	tapentadol	PENTAZOCINE	NALOXONE
CODEINE	tramadol	buprenorphine	NALTREXONE
FENTANYL		butorphanol	nalmefene
HEROIN		dezocine	alvimopan
hydrocodone		nalbuphine	methylnaltrexone
hydromorphone			
levorphanol			
MEPERIDINE			
METHADONE			
MORPHINE			
oxycodone			
oxymorphone			
propoxyphene			
remifentanil			
sufentanil			

ACTIONS OF MORPHINE AND THE OTHER AGONISTS

Morphine causes
  1. Analgesia
  2. Respiratory depression
  3. Spasm of smooth muscle of the gastrointestinal (GI) and genitourinary (GU) tracts, including the biliary tract
  4. Pinpoint pupils

Morphine has actions in many organ systems. These actions are sometimes used for therapeutic purposes and sometimes are considered side effects. Therefore, learning the important actions means that you have learned both therapeutic uses and adverse effects at one time.

CNS: In most people morphine produces drowsiness and sedation in addition to the reduction in awareness of pain. Initial doses of morphine often cause nausea, more often in ambulatory patients than in those who are bedridden. This effect is due to direct stimulation of the chemoreceptor trigger zone in the medulla oblongata and to an increase in vestibular sensitivity.

Morphine is an effective cough suppressant because it has a direct effect in the medulla. Morphine is not used for this purpose, but codeine (another agonist) is frequently prescribed for its cough suppressive action.

EYE: Morphine produces pupillary constriction by a direct action in the brainstem nucleus of the oculomotor nerve (Edinger-Westphal). This is the classic pinpoint pupil that you will hear mentioned in the emergency room.

RESPIRATORY: Morphine depresses all phases of respiratory activity through an action in the CNS. The hypoxic drive for breathing is also depressed.

CARDIOVASCULAR (CV): Morphine has essentially no effect on the cardiovascular system at therapeutic doses.

GASTROINTESTINAL (GI): Morphine increases the resting tone of the smooth muscle of the entire GI tract. This results in a decrease in the movement of stomach and intestinal contents, which may lead to spasm (pain) and to constipation. Morphine also produces spasm of the smooth muscle of the biliary tract. Tolerance does not develop to the constipating action. Two μ-receptor antagonists that do not cross the blood–brain barrier (alvimopan and methylnaltrexone) can be used to relieve the constipation.

GENITOURINARY (GU): Similar to its action on the GI tract, morphine increases the tone and produces spasm of the smooth muscle in the GU tract. This can lead to urinary retention.

> Withdrawal from narcotics in a dependent person consists of autonomic hyperactivity, such as diarrhea, vomiting, chills, fever, tearing, and runny nose. Tremor, abdominal cramps, and pain can be severe.

That was a quick summary of the most important information about morphine's actions. If you are doing well up to this point, continue and learn some specific details of some of the agonists. If you have some trouble with the preceding details, review the next section on another pass through the material.

DISTINGUISHING FEATURES OF SOME AGONISTS

> CODEINE is used for suppressing cough and for pain. It is much less potent than morphine.

> HEROIN is more lipid soluble than morphine and, therefore, rapidly crosses the blood–brain barrier. It is hydrolyzed to morphine in the brain; thus, it is a prodrug.

> MEPERIDINE is less potent than morphine and less spasmogenic. It has no cough suppressive ability.

Here are a few more things that you may need to know. Meperidine is also used in obstetrics. Unlike morphine, meperidine produces no more respiratory depression in the fetus than in the mother.

Diphenoxylate and loperamide (relatives of meperidine) are used to treat diarrhea, in part because they are not absorbed from the GI tract.

> FENTANYL, sufentanil, alfentanil and remifentanil (IV only) are much more potent than morphine but have short durations of action. They are used (mostly) in anesthesiology.

> METHADONE is a highly effective analgesic after oral administration and has a much longer duration of action than morphine.

Methadone (an agonist) is used in the treatment of patients addicted to narcotics, which may seem counterintuitive. Use of an antagonist would put an addict into immediate and frightening withdrawal. Replacement of an addict's heroin with a long-acting oral agonist reduces cravings, prevents withdrawal, and allows behavioral modification. Buprenorphine is also used to treat opiate addiction.

> The weak agonist/reuptake inhibitors are μ-agonists and norepinephrine (and serotonin) reuptake inhibitors.

Opiates are often used in combination with the non-opiate analgesics (aspirin and acetaminophen).

OPIOID ANTAGONISTS

> Opioid antagonists have no effect when administered alone. When given after a dose of agonist, they promptly reverse all of the actions of the agonist.

This is basically the definition of an antagonist from general principles.

> NALOXONE is the *drug of choice* for narcotic overdose.

OPIOID AGONIST-ANTAGONISTS

These drugs appear to be agonists at the κ receptor, which gives them analgesic activity. They are also antagonists at the μ receptor. This leads to their classification as mixed agonist-antagonists.

> PENTAZOCINE produces effects that are qualitatively similar to morphine.

> PENTAZOCINE causes acute withdrawal in patients who have received regular doses of morphine or other agonists.

General Anesthetics

- Organization of Class
- Uptake and Distribution of Inhalational Anesthetics
- Elimination of Inhalational Anesthetics
- Potency of General Anesthetics
- Specific Gases and Volatile Liquids
- Specific Intravenous Agents

ORGANIZATION OF CLASS

The state of general anesthesia is a drug-induced absence of perception of all sensations. Depths of anesthesia appropriate for surgical procedures can be achieved with a wide variety of drugs. General anesthetics are administered primarily by inhalation and intravenous (IV) injection. These routes of administration allow control of the dosage and time course of action.

For these drugs, understanding the principles of uptake, distribution, and elimination are the major focus, particularly for the inhaled anesthetics. The mechanism of action of most of the anesthetics is unknown. You should be able to recognize the names of the general anesthetics and know a few specific facts about these drugs (Figure 25–1).

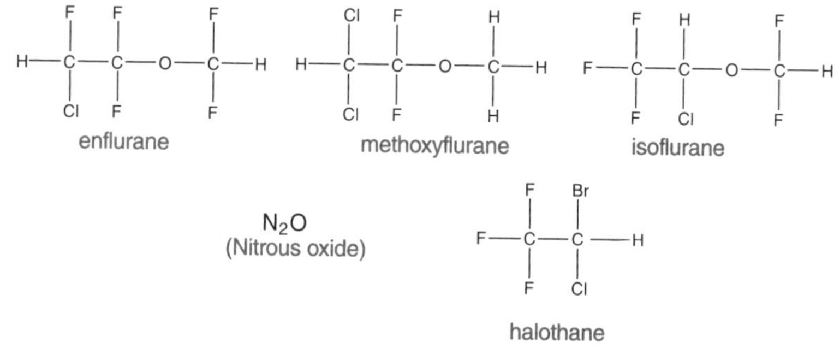

FIGURE 25–1 Structures of some of the inhalational drugs. Notice the very simple structures and the presence of fluoride.

Inhaled Drugs	IV Drugs
desflurane	PROPOFOL
ENFLURANE	THIOPENTAL
HALOTHANE	etomidate
ISOFLURANE	ketamine
NITROUS OXIDE	
sevoflurane	

UPTAKE AND DISTRIBUTION OF INHALATIONAL ANESTHETICS

The tension of a gas in a mixture is proportional to its concentration. Therefore, the terms *tension* and *concentration* are often used interchangeably. The term *partial pressure* is also used interchangeably with tension.

> When a constant tension (concentration) of anesthetic gas is inhaled, the tension (concentration) in arterial blood approaches that of the agent in the inspired mixture. The tension (concentration) in the brain is always approaching the tension (concentration) in arterial blood.

The level of general anesthesia is dependent on the concentration of anesthetic in the brain.

> The solubility of an agent is expressed as the blood–gas partition coefficient.

The blood–gas partition coefficient represents the ratio of anesthetic concentration in blood to the concentration in the gas phase. The blood–gas coefficient is high for very soluble agents and low for relatively insoluble anesthetics such as nitrous oxide.

> The more soluble an anesthetic is in blood, the more of it must be dissolved in blood to raise its partial pressure in the blood.

The potential reservoir for relatively soluble gases is large and will be filled more slowly. Therefore, for soluble gases the rate at which the tension (partial pressure) in the arterial blood approaches the inspired partial pressure is slow. Also, the rate at which the brain partial pressure approaches the arterial partial pressure is slow. The opposite is true for more insoluble anesthetics.

> The speed of onset of anesthesia is inversely related to the solubility of the gas in blood:
>   More soluble (high blood–gas partition coefficient) = Slower onset
>   Less soluble (low blood–gas partition coefficient) = Faster onset

Onset of anesthesia is also related to pulmonary ventilation, rate of pulmonary blood flow, tissue blood flow, and solubility of the gas in the tissues.

ELIMINATION OF INHALATIONAL ANESTHETICS

> Elimination of anesthetics is influenced by pulmonary ventilation, blood flow, and solubility of the gas.

The major factors that affect the rate of elimination of the anesthetics are the same factors that are important in the uptake phase. This makes these principles easy to remember.

Most of the inhaled anesthetics are eliminated unchanged in the exhaled gas. A small percentage of the anesthetics are metabolized in the liver. It has been suggested that the production of a toxic metabolite may be responsible for most of the hepatic and renal toxicities observed with these agents. One example of this is methoxyflurane. It has been associated with renal failure as a result of the toxic amounts of fluoride ions that are produced when the drug is metabolized. More details about this process are available in your pharmacology textbook.

POTENCY OF GENERAL ANESTHETICS

Anesthesiologists have accepted a measure of potency for the inhalational anesthetics known as the minimum alveolar concentration (MAC).

> Minimum alveolar concentration (MAC) is defined as the alveolar concentration at one atmosphere that produces immobility in 50% of patients exposed to a painful stimulus.

The MAC is usually expressed as the percentage of gas in the mixture required to achieve immobility in 50% of patients exposed to a painful stimulus. The alveolar concentration is used for this definition because the concentration in the lung can be easily and accurately measured. The real concentration that we would want to know is the brain concentration. It is not so easy to measure brain levels, but we know that brain levels are directly correlated to alveolar levels. So, the MAC is a good approximation of brain levels.

SPECIFIC GASES AND VOLATILE LIQUIDS

Each of these drugs has a whole range of effects on the lungs, heart, and circulation. It is probably advisable to read through a detailed description of these effects and pick out some trends to memorize.

> NITROUS OXIDE is a relatively insoluble gas, with an MAC of about 105% that has little effect on blood pressure or respiration. It does produce analgesia.

The low solubility means that onset of anesthesia with nitrous oxide is very fast. The MAC indicates that nitrous oxide has very low potency—so low in fact, that more than 100% of the inspired gas needs to be nitrous oxide to produce immobility in 50% of patients exposed to a painful stimulus. That is why nitrous oxide is used in combination with other agents.

SPECIFIC INTRAVENOUS AGENTS

Some barbiturates (thiopental and methohexital) and benzodiazepines (midazolam) are used for anesthesia, particularly during induction. They are covered in Chapter 19. Thus, for our purposes here, it is just a matter of adding what you already know about barbiturates and benzodiazepines to these names and associating them with anesthesia. These drugs do not produce analgesia.

The majority of IV drugs used to induce anesthesia are slowly metabolized and excreted and depend on redistribution to terminate their pharmacological effects.

> PROPOFOL and etomidate are two drugs used intravenously to produce general anesthesia.

Propofol (milk of anesthesia) is administered intravenously and is often used for short out-patient surgeries or procedures.

On your first pass, you should recognize these names and know that they are general anesthetics. On the second pass, you should try to add some details about analgesia and cardiovascular effects.

Local Anesthetics

Organization of Class
Mechanism of Action
Special Features about Individual Agents

ORGANIZATION OF CLASS

These drugs are applied locally and block nerve conduction. Nerve fibers are not affected equally. Loss of sympathetic function occurs first, followed by loss of pin-prick sensation and temperature, and finally, motor function. The effect of local anesthetics is reversible: their use is followed by complete recovery of nerve function with no evidence of structural damage.

All the local anesthetics consist of a hydrophilic amino group linked through a connecting group of variable length to a lipophilic aromatic portion (benzene ring, Figure 26–1). In the intermediate chain, there is either an ester linkage or an amide linkage.

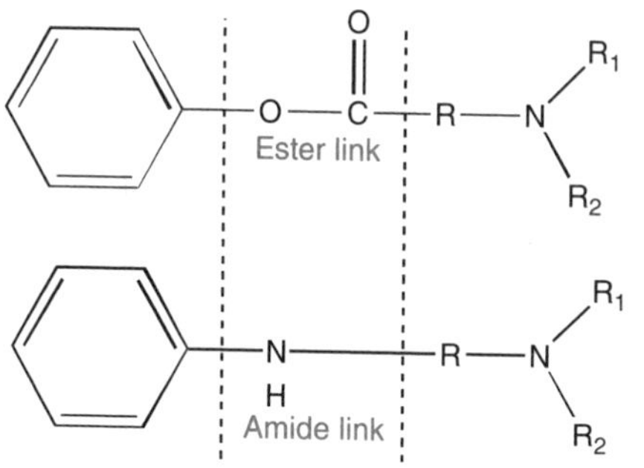

FIGURE 26–1 Main structures of the ester and amide local anesthetics.

The commonly used local anesthetics can be classified as esters or amides based on the linkage in this intermediate chain. It is not *as* important to know which drugs are esters and which are amides, as it is to know that there *is* a difference. The amide local anesthetics are chemically stable *in vivo*, whereas the esters are rapidly hydrolyzed by plasma cholinesterase. One interesting, but trivial, fact is that metabolism of the ester local anesthetics leads to formation of para-amino-benzoic acid (PABA), which is thought to be allergenic.

ESTERS	AMIDES	
COCAINE	LIDOCAINE	ropivacaine
PROCAINE	bupivacaine	articaine
benzocaine	etidocaine	levobupivacaine
chloroprocaine	mepivacaine	
tetracaine	prilocaine	

The "-caine" ending on each of these drug names tells you that they are local anesthetics.

> Adverse effects of the local anesthetics result from systemic absorption of toxic amounts of the drugs.

Death can occur from respiratory failure secondary to medullary depression or from hypotension and cardiovascular collapse.

MECHANISM OF ACTION

> Local anesthetics block the sodium channel in the nerve membrane.

Application of a local anesthetic inhibits the inward movement of Na^+ ions. This results in elevation of the threshold for electrical excitation, reduction in the rate of rise of the action potential and slowing of the propagation of the impulse. At high enough concentrations, the local anesthetics completely block conduction of impulses down the nerve.

For those of you interested in this area, there is a fascinating story relating pH to ionization of the local anesthetics to drug action. For details, see your textbook.

Some local anesthetics have a vasodilator effect resulting in termination of their action. For these anesthetics, a small amount of a vasoconstrictor can be added to the injection. This leads to increased duration of action, reduction in risk of systemic toxicity, and lessens bleeding locally. Epinephrine is the most common vasoconstrictor. Epinephrine-containing solutions are not injected into tissues supplied by end arteries, such as the fingers, toes, ears, nose, or penis.

SPECIAL FEATURES ABOUT INDIVIDUAL AGENTS

> LIDOCAINE is a local anesthetic also used intravenously in the treatment of cardiac arrhythmias.

> COCAINE is better known as a drug of abuse, but it is also an effective local anesthetic (think ENT).

PART V Chemotherapeutic Agents

CHAPTER 27:   Introduction to Chemotherapy   137

CHAPTER 28:   Inhibitors of Cell Wall Synthesis   142

CHAPTER 29:   Protein Synthesis Inhibitors   149

CHAPTER 30:   Folate Antagonists   154

CHAPTER 31:   Quinolones and Urinary Tract Antiseptics   156

CHAPTER 32:   Drugs Used in Tuberculosis and Leprosy   158

CHAPTER 33:   Antifungal Drugs   162

CHAPTER 34:   Anthelmintic Drugs   166

CHAPTER 35:   Antiviral Drugs   169

CHAPTER 36:   Antiprotozoal Drugs   175

CHAPTER 37:   Anticancer Drugs   179

Introduction to Chemotherapy

Approach to the Antimicrobials
General Principles of Therapy
Definitions
Important Concepts to Understand
Classification of Antimicrobials

APPROACH TO THE ANTIMICROBIALS

Students often have difficulty with the antibiotics, not because of any difficult concepts but because of the large number of drugs in this class. It can also be overwhelming to try to memorize the organisms that are sensitive to each drug.

Try this approach. First, make absolutely sure that you understand the general principles of therapy and some definitions. We'll go over these in this chapter.

Second, be aware of the classes of antibiotics and the mechanism of action for the class. Note any features that are common to all drugs in the class.

Third, learn the particular adverse effects or special features of administration for the drugs in the class. Do any of the drugs cause potentially *fatal* side effects?

Fourth, learn the broad categories of bacterial spectrum and whether any of the drugs in the class are the *drug of choice* for the treatment of a particular organism. For example, are the drugs good against all of the gram-positive bacteria, but none of the gram negative? It may be useful to quickly review the most common bacteria at this point. Can you say which bacteria are gram positive and which are gram negative? A solid knowledge of this content will really help when you try to learn about antibiotics. Remember that the sensitivity of bacteria to antibiotics changes over time and in different locations.

This looks like a long list of things to learn, but it is really quite manageable. Don't get too bogged down in trying to remember the second-line drugs for treatment of certain organisms or which drug to use in case of allergies, and so on. This can be added later to the base of knowledge that you develop now.

GENERAL PRINCIPLES OF THERAPY

To be a useful antibiotic, a compound should inhibit the growth of bacteria without harming the human host.

This should be self-evident, but it is the basis for understanding most of the mechanisms of action of these drugs. The compound should affect some aspect of bacteria that is not present in mammalian cells. We'll come back to that later.

> The drug should penetrate body tissues in order to reach the bacteria.

This again should be self-evident. Again, this is the basis for knowing whether a drug is orally absorbed and whether it will cross the blood-brain barrier. For example, if the patient has a gastrointestinal (GI) infection, you would give a drug orally that is not absorbed by the GI tract. The bacteria are thus treated, and the patient has few side effects. Likewise, the drugs that are used to treat meningitis are ones that cross the blood-brain barrier. The drug that is extremely effective against *Haemophilus influenzae* does no good for the patient if it cannot reach the organisms.

DEFINITIONS

> *Spectrum*—as in narrow, broad, and extended—is a term used to convey an impression of the range of bacteria that a drug is effective against.

Drugs are designated as narrow spectrum if they are only effective against one class of bacteria. They are designated as broad spectrum if they are effective against a range of bacteria. If a narrow-spectrum agent is modified chemically (as in adding a new side chain), and the new compound is effective against more bacteria than the parent compound, then the new drug is said to have an extended spectrum. This is easy enough.

> Bacteriostatic versus bactericidal—be sure you know the difference.

Textbooks often place a lot of emphasis on whether a drug will arrest the growth and replication of a bacteria (-static) or actually kill the bacteria (-cidal). If a drug is bacteriostatic, the patient's immune system must complete the task of clearing the body of the invaders. However, these terms are relative and not always accurate. Some drugs can kill one type of bug (-cidal) and only arrest the growth of another (-static). So, don't focus too much time on this early on.

IMPORTANT CONCEPTS TO UNDERSTAND

> Resistance of bacteria to an antibiotic can occur by mutation, adaptation, or gene transfer.

The whole area of bacterial resistance has received much attention and appropriately so. Many bacteria are becoming resistant to the available drugs. Students need to have some idea of the mechanisms of bacterial resistance.

Bacteria undergo spontaneous mutation at a frequency of about 1 in 10^{16} cells. Mutation may make bacteria resistant to an antibiotic, or it may not.

Adaptation can take several routes. The bacteria may alter the uptake of the drug by changes in their lipopolysaccharide coat. Or they may improve a transport system that removes the drug from the cell. The bacteria may increase metabolism through a pathway that bypasses the effect of the antibiotic.

Gene transfer occurs through plasmids and transposons. Plasmids are extrachromosomal genetic elements (pieces of RNA or DNA that are not part of chromosomes). These may code for enzymes that inactivate antimicrobials. The plasmids are transferred from bacteria to bacteria by conjugation and transduction.

Transposons are segments of genetic material with insertion sequences. They are incorporated into the genetic makeup of bacteria and can carry code for enzymes that inactivate the antimicrobials.

> Adverse effects can be allergic, toxic, idiosyncratic, or related to changes in the normal body flora.

Adverse effects of antibiotics are grouped into general categories. The first three categories (allergic, toxic, and idiosyncratic) apply to all drugs. The last (changes in normal body flora) is unique to antibiotics.

A reminder: Idiosyncratic reactions are reactions that are not related to immune responses or known drug properties. Examples of idiosyncratic reactions include the hemolysis that occurs in glucose-6-phosphate dehydrogenase (G-6-PD)–deficient patients after treatment with sulfonamides, and the peripheral neuropathy that develops after isoniazid administration in genetically slow acetylators.

The phrase "alterations in the normal body flora" usually refers to changes that occur within the GI tract. Normally the gut is host to friendly bacteria that help in the digestion of the food we eat. If an antimicrobial agent is given orally, it may kill these friendly bacteria. Other bacteria that are resistant to the antimicrobial can then overgrow and repopulate the GI tract. This secondary infection is sometimes called a superinfection. The most common example is the overgrowth of *Clostridium difficile*. It produces a toxin that causes a disorder called pseudomembranous colitis. As you read in your textbook, you will probably see comments about the incidence of colitis after use of a particular antibiotic.

> Combinations of antimicrobial agents can take advantage of the mechanisms of action to produce a synergistic effect.

The area of drug combinations is where an understanding of the mechanisms of action of the antimicrobials becomes important. You can combine agents with different sites of action.

Example: Combine a protein synthesis inhibitor (these are bacteriostatic; that is, they stop cell growth) with a drug that affects cell wall synthesis (which requires the cell to be dividing to have an action). Does this combination make sense?

This combination does not make sense. The protein synthesis inhibitor will stop cell growth and prevent cell division so that the second drug will have no effect (except possible side effects).

Example: Two drugs both inhibit production of a key metabolic product, but at two different sites in the metabolic pathway. Does this combination make sense?

This combination is useful. The two drugs, trimethoprim and sulfamethoxazole, inhibit the synthesis of folic acid at different steps in the pathway. They, in a sense, help each other out.

Example: The combination of a cell wall synthesis inhibitor and a drug that needs to act intracellularly. Does this combination make sense?

This combination is extremely useful. It describes the combination of penicillins and aminoglycosides. The penicillins alter the cell wall and enhance the penetration of the aminoglycoside.

> Culture and sensitivity testing will determine the minimum inhibitory concentration (MIC) for the bacteria.

The best way to determine the proper antimicrobial agent for a patient is to culture and identify the organism. The laboratory can then run a test for sensitivity of the organism to a series of antimicrobials. They can determine the minimum inhibitory concentration (MIC), which is the lowest concentration of the drug that inhibits growth of the organism. The drug to which the organism is most sensitive has the lowest MIC. Culture and sensitivity (C and S) testing is extremely useful in the selection of the best antimicrobial agent to use but it can take several days, depending on the growth rate of the organism.

> Dosing schedules for antibiotics depend on whether the antibiotic action is time dependent or concentration dependent and whether the drug has a postantibiotic effect.

Some classes of antimicrobial drugs are most effect when the concentration of the drug stays above the MIC (time dependent). For these drugs increasing the dose to get a higher maximal concentration does not improve the effect and can increase the adverse effects. For other antibiotics, the peak concentration is the most important for determining the effect (concentration dependent). An antibiotic is said to have a post-antibiotic effect, when it continues to be effective even though the plasma concentration has fallen below the MIC.

Now let's look at the specific drugs.

CLASSIFICATION OF ANTIMICROBIALS

Antimicrobial Drug Classes
Inhibitors of cell wall synthesis
β-Lactams
Others
Protein synthesis inhibitors
Folate antagonists
Quinolones and other drugs

Notice how your textbook organizes these drugs. Some books focus primarily on structure and others primarily on mechanisms. Don't let this confuse you. There are two really big groups of drugs: the cell wall synthesis inhibitors and the protein synthesis inhibitors. This is in part because bacteria have a cell wall, whereas mammalian cells do not. Also, bacteria have different ribosomal units than mammalian cells. Therefore, targeting cell wall or protein synthesis kills the bacteria and not the host.

CHAPTER
28 Inhibitors of Cell Wall Synthesis

General Features
β-Lactams
    Penicillins
    Cephalosporins
    Carbapenems
    Monobactams (Aztreonam)
Other Inhibitors of Cell Wall Synthesis
    Glycopeptides
    Bacitracin
    Fosfomycin
    Daptomycin

GENERAL FEATURES

> These drugs all work by inhibiting the synthesis of the bacterial cell wall.

You probably guessed this from the title of the chapter. However, this is a real key point. If you can remember this, you are well on your way to learning these drugs.

The final step in the synthesis of the bacterial cell wall is a cross-linking of adjacent peptidoglycan strands by a process called *transpeptidation*. The penicillins and cephalosporins are structurally similar to the terminal portion of the peptidoglycan strands and can compete for and bind to the enzymes that catalyze transpeptidation and cross-linking. These enzymes are called penicillin-binding proteins (PBPs). Interference with these enzymes results in the formation of a structurally weakened cell wall, oddly shaped bacteria, and ultimately, death.

Now, let's divide the cell wall synthesis inhibitors into two groups based on chemical structure: β-lactams and others.

β-LACTAMS

> β-Lactam antibiotics are best against rapidly growing organisms. They are not effective against intracellular organisms.

This is where your knowledge of the microbes can really help you. β-Lactam antibiotics interfere with the synthesis of the cell wall, which is on the outside of the bacteria. Rapidly growing bacteria are making lots of cell walls making them susceptible to these antibiotics.

> All of the drugs in this group contain a β-lactam ring in their structure.

Normally, we do not worry too much about the structures of drugs, but in this case we make an important exception. These drugs are often referred to as the β-lactam group. This is because they all have a β-lactam ring in their chemical structure, and it is this β-lactam ring that makes them effective antimicrobials.

> Some bacteria inactivate β-lactam antibiotics by an enzyme that opens the β-lactam ring.

Some bacteria contain an enzyme, called *β-lactamase*, that can open the β-lactam ring (Figure 28–1). This leads to inactivation of the antibiotic. The most common mode of drug resistance is plasmid transfer of the genetic code for the β-lactamase enzyme. There is a β-lactamase specific for the penicillins—it is called *penicillinase*—and a β-lactamase specific for the cephalosporins—it is called *cephalosporinase*. Inactivation of these drugs by β-lactamases is a major problem and has been the focus of intense research.

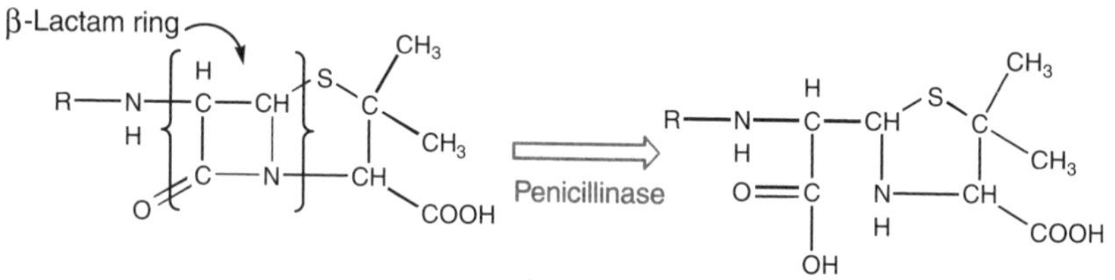

FIGURE 28–1 Here we can see the lactam ring and its opening by penicillinase.

> The inactivation of these drugs by β-lactamases can be dealt with by two approaches:
> 1. Give a β-lactamase inhibitor at the same time.
> 2. Make chemical modifications in the structure of the drug to make it more resistant to inactivation.

> CLAVULANIC ACID and SULBACTAM are β-lactamase inhibitors that are given together with β-lactam drugs to increase their effectiveness.

One way to increase the effectiveness of β-lactam antibiotics is to give a β-lactamase inhibitor at the same time. The most commonly used ones are clavulanic acid and sulbactam. You may also come across tazobactam or avibactam.

The other approach is to chemically modify the structure of the compounds to make the β-lactam ring more difficult for the enzyme to open.

You now know a lot about penicillins and cephalosporins, and we haven't even listed them yet. See? This is really not too difficult.

PENICILLINS

Most books divide penicillins into three or four groups. The naturally occurring ones are those that are made by the mold. The rest are chemical modifications of these original penicillins to try to improve the bacterial spectrum and improve resistance to the penicillinase (β-lactamase).

Penicillin Type	Spectrum
Natural	
PENICILLIN G	Narrow spectrum (gram-positive);
PENICILLIN V	penicillinase sensitive
benzathine pen G	
Penicillinase resistant	
methicillin	Narrow spectrum (gram-positive);
cloxacillin	synthesized to be penicillinase resistant
dicloxacillin	
nafcillin	
oxacillin	
Aminopenicillins	
AMOXICILLIN	Broad spectrum (some gram-negative activity also);
AMPICILLIN	penicillinase sensitive
Extended spectrum	
azlocillin	Active against *Pseudomonas;* relatively
carbenicillin	ineffective against gram-positive organisms
mezlocillin	
PIPERACILLIN	
ticarcillin	

First of all, notice that penicillins are easy to identify by the "-cillin" ending. The first group contains the G and V penicillins. The second group contains the three *oxa*cillins. The third group starts with "am-" for amino group. Except for methicillin (discontinued in the United States) and nafcillin, the rest are in the last group. In the "extended spectrum" group, only piperacillin is in use in the United States. Again, this is really not too hard. Keep them categorized and remember the general outline for the spectrum and you'll do just fine.

The oral absorption of the penicillins is poor; however, there are exceptions. If you have time and energy, you can learn the orally active ones. Most of these only cross the blood–brain barrier if it is inflamed. If you have a bit more time, add the ones that can be used in meningitis.

> Penicillins are excreted by tubular secretion that can be blocked by probenecid.

Penicillins are, for the most part, excreted by active tubular secretion. Blocking tubular secretion is a relatively simple way to prolong the action of the drug. Probenecid can be administered along with the penicillins, and it blocks the tubular secretion.

> The most important adverse effect of penicillins as a group is hypersensitivity reaction. It can be *fatal*.

All penicillins can give rise to allergic reactions. These reactions have been divided into three types: immediate, accelerated, and late. The immediate is the most severe.

The immediate reaction occurs within 20 minutes after parenteral administration and consists of apprehension, itching (pruritus), paresthesia (numbness and tingling), wheezing, choking, fever, edema, and generalized urticaria (hives). It can lead to hypotension, shock, loss of consciousness, and death. The immediate hypersensitivity reaction to penicillin appears to be mediated by immunoglobulin E (IgE) antibodies to the minor determinants.

The accelerated reaction appears 1 to 72 hours after drug administration, and it consists mainly of urticaria (hives). The late reaction is more common with the semisynthetics and appears 72 hours to several weeks after drug administration. It consists mainly of skin rashes.

> Penicillins do not get into the brain unless there is inflammation. They typically have short half-lives and are often used in combination with aminoglycosides.

CEPHALOSPORINS

These drugs are classified into generations. It is impossible to learn all the names (but they almost all begin with "cef" or "ceph"), so focus on the differences between the generations and try to learn three names in each generation. I have listed just the more common ones.

Cephalosporin Type	Spectrum
First generation	Narrow spectrum similar to broad spectrum
CEFAZOLIN	penicillins; sensitive to β-lactamases
CEPHALEXIN	

(Continued)

Cephalosporin Type	Spectrum
Second generation	Increased activity toward gram-negative organisms;
CEFACLOR	increased stability
CEFAMANDOLE	
CEFOXITIN	
Third generation	Even broader in spectrum and more resistant
CEFOTAXIME	to β-lactamases
CEFTAZIDIME	
CEFTRIAXONE	
Fourth generation	Gram-positive and gram-negative activity, especially
cefepime	against *Pseudomonas aeruginosa;* includes gram-negative
cefpirome	organisms with multiple-drug resistance patterns

Believe it or not, this is most of what you need to know. Add a few facts about absorption, distribution, and elimination and you'll be doing great.

Some of these drugs can be given orally (such as cephalexin and cefaclor). You can learn these if you want to try.

The third-generation cephalosporins are used extensively in the treatment and prophylaxis of infections in hospitalized patients. The fourth-generation drugs are being designed to target organisms with multiple-drug resistance.

These drugs are relatively nontoxic. Here are a few facts to consider learning:

1. There is some cross-allergy with penicillins.
2. Some cephalosporins have anti–vitamin K effects (bleeding).
3. Some cephalosporins can cause a disulfiram-like reaction because they block alcohol oxidation, causing acetaldehyde to accumulate.

There is a drug related to the cephalosporins, loracarbef, which is only mentioned here because of the quite different name. You should learn its name with the other cephalosporins, even though technically it is in a different class (the carbacephems).

CARBAPENEMS

This class of β-lactam antibiotics contains imipenem, doripenem, ertapenem, and meropenem. All are administered intravenously.

> IMIPENEM with CILASTATIN is a broad-spectrum β-lactam antibiotic.

Imipenem is the antibiotic. It is hydrolyzed by a renal dipeptidase on the luminal brush border of proximal tubular epithelium (i.e., in the kidney) to a somewhat toxic metabolite that is inactive as an antimicrobial. Cilastatin inhibits the renal dipeptidase. Therefore, the two compounds are always administered together. Meropenem is more stable to the renal peptidase and does not need the co-administration of cilastin. Note the common "penem" ending of each name.

MONOBACTAMS (AZTREONAM)

The term *monobactam* refers to the chemical structure of this class of β-lactams. The only one currently available is aztreonam.

> AZTREONAM is an excellent drug for aerobic gram-negative bacteria, including *Pseudomonas*, but it is ineffective against gram-positive organisms and anaerobes.

Aztreonam is an example of a narrow-spectrum drug and is highly resistant to the action of β-lactamases. It has an unusual spectrum, especially compared to other β-lactams, so it is a good idea to file this one away in your memory bank.

OTHER INHIBITORS OF CELL WALL SYNTHESIS

These last few drugs are inhibitors of cell wall synthesis but are not β-lactam compounds.

GLYCOPEPTIDES

Vancomycin, dalbavancin, oritavancin, teicoplanin, and telavancin are glycopeptides that inhibit cell wall synthesis by preventing polymerization of the linear peptidoglycans. Note the "-vancin" endings.

> VANCOMYCIN is only effective against the gram-positive organisms. It is very poorly absorbed orally but can be used orally for treatment of *Clostridium difficile* colitis.

Vancomycin can cause a dose-related ototoxicity that produces tinnitus (ringing), high-tone deafness, hearing loss, and possible deafness. This is serious enough to commit to memory. Vancomycin has also caused a condition called "red man syndrome" that is due to histamine release with a fast drug infusion.

BACITRACIN

> Bacitracin is a mixture of polypeptides that inhibit cell wall synthesis. It is used topically.

Bacitracin binds to a lipid carrier that transports cell wall precursors to the growing cell wall. Therefore, it can be classified as a cell wall synthesis inhibitor. Because bacitracin has serious nephrotoxicity, it is only used topically.

FOSFOMYCIN

Fosfomycin inhibits one of the first steps in the synthesis of peptidoglycan (i.e., the cell wall) by inhibiting the enzyme enolpyruvyl transferase. It is used for the treatment of uncomplicated urinary tract infections.

DAPTOMYCIN

Daptomycin is a lipopeptide antibiotic with a spectrum of activity similar to vancomycin. It binds to the membrane of the bacteria and causes a depolarization of the bacteria. This loss of membrane potential results in bacterial death. So, it is not really an inhibitor of cell wall synthesis, but function.

CHAPTER

29

Protein Synthesis Inhibitors

General Features
Aminoglycosides
Tetracyclines
Macrolides
Streptogramins and Oxazolidinones
Chloramphenicol
Clindamycin

GENERAL FEATURES

Protein synthesis machinery, including ribosomes, is somewhat different in bacteria compared to mammalian cells. This accounts for the selectivity of this group of drugs for bacteria. Some textbooks and instructors make a point of having students know which ribosomal subunit a class of drugs binds to. However, this is not of primary importance. If you already know it, try not to forget it. If you are struggling with the antimicrobials at this point, save this fact for later. These drugs require binding to an intracellular protein (ribosomal subunit). Therefore, the drugs need to gain entry into the cell. A major route of resistance for the bacteria is to block the movement of the drugs into the cell.

For the protein synthesis inhibitors, the class names are related to the chemical structure of the compounds in each group, but don't worry too much about remembering the class name. It is more important to know the individual drug names here.

AMINOGLYCOSIDES

The aminoglycosides are broad-spectrum antimicrobials. However, anaerobic bacteria are generally resistant to them.

Some bacteria use an oxygen-dependent transport system to bring the aminoglycosides into the cell. The anaerobes (with non–oxygen-based metabolism) do not have this system. Therefore, they are generally resistant to the aminoglycosides.

149

- GENTAMICIN
- TOBRAMYCIN
- amikacin
- neomycin
- streptomycin

Notice that the names of the aminoglycosides all end in "-mycin" or "-micin," except amikacin. However, the drug companies have thrown a curve ball here, because the drug clindamycin and all the macrolides (erythromycin, clarithromycin, etc.) also end in "-mycin." So take a moment to compare the list of names here with the one included later in the chapter. Be sure that you can recognize which class a particular name belongs to.

> Aminoglycosides are poorly absorbed from the gastrointestinal (GI) tract and none cross the blood-brain barrier.

Most aminoglycosides must be administered parenterally. They are highly polar compounds and are relatively insoluble in fat. They do not readily penetrate most cells without help from penicillins or a transport system.

Recall the synergism between penicillins and aminoglycosides that was mentioned in the introduction to chemotherapy (see Chapter 27). The penicillins cause cell wall abnormalities that allow the aminoglycosides to gain entry into the bacteria.

> Aminoglycosides have ototoxicity, nephrotoxicity, and neuromuscular toxicity.

The margin of safety with these drugs is small. This means that the toxic concentration is only slightly higher than the therapeutic concentration.

The ototoxicity can be both cochlear (auditory) and vestibular. The symptoms include tinnitus (ringing), deafness, vertigo or unsteadiness of gait, and high-frequency hearing loss. The cochlear toxicity results from selective destruction of the outer hair cells in the organ of Corti.

The nephrotoxicity is related to the rapid uptake of the drug by proximal tubular cells. The proximal tubular cells are then killed. Acute nephrotoxicity is reversible.

The neurotoxicity is caused by the blockade of presynaptic release of acetylcholine at the neuromuscular junction. There is also some postsynaptic blockade as well. This leads to weakness and can lead to respiratory depression.

TETRACYCLINES

- TETRACYCLINE
- demeclocycline
- DOXYCYCLINE
- minocycline
- omadacycline

These drug names are easy to recognize, because they all end in "-cycline." Similar to the aminoglycosides, the tetracyclines accumulate in the cytoplasm by an energy-dependent transport system. This transport system is not present in mammalian cells. Resistance to tetracyclines occurs when bacteria mutate in a way that makes them unable to accumulate the drug.

> Tetracyclines are broad-spectrum antibiotics and are bacteriostatic.

Tetracyclines are useful in the treatment of gram-positive and gram-negative facultative organisms and anaerobes.

> Tetracyclines have also found use in rickettsial diseases (Rocky Mountain spotted fever), chlamydial diseases, cholera, Lyme disease (spirochetes), and mycoplasma pneumonia.

Notice that tetracyclines are useful in the treatment of some oddball diseases, particularly the rickettsiae and spirochetes.

> Food impairs the absorption of the tetracyclines.

Except for doxycycline and minocycline, food impairs the absorption of the tetracyclines. The tetracyclines form insoluble chelates with calcium, magnesium, and other metals. The use of antacids when taking tetracyclines is therefore not advised.

> Tetracyclines are associated with staining of the teeth, retardation of bone growth, and photosensitivity.

The major side effects of the tetracyclines are related to their incorporation into teeth and bone. They cause the teeth to be discolored and can retard bone growth. For these reasons, they are not recommended for use in children or pregnant women. There is an increased incidence of an abnormal sunburn reaction in people taking tetracyclines (photosensitivity).

Glycylcyclines are derivatives of the tetracyclines, and they also work by inhibiting protein synthesis. Tigecycline is the first drug available in this class.

MACROLIDES

- ERYTHROMYCIN
- azithromycin
- clarithromycin

These names are easy to recognize because they all end in "-thromycin." Thus, they should be readily distinguishable from the aminoglycosides that end in "-mycin." Erythromycin and its relatives are generally well absorbed orally.

> Erythromycin and its relatives are of particular use in the treatment of patients with *Mycoplasma* infections, pneumonia, Legionnaires disease, chlamydial infections, diphtheria, and pertussis.

Books vary somewhat as to their designation of erythromycin as the *drug of choice* for some of these diseases. Check your textbook or class notes and highlight those diseases that you need to know. Notice that many of these fall into the category of oddball infections.

Compare and contrast the tetracyclines and erythromycin. One mnemonic that is sometimes used to remember the organisms for which erythromycin is the drug of choice is Legionnaires Camp on My Border (*Legionella, Campylobacter, Mycoplasma, Bordetella*).

The macrolides have few serious side effects—none that deserve a box of their own. GI upset is common, but you would have guessed that one, right?

There is a related group of antibiotics, the ketolides, that were derived from the macrolides. The first is telithromycin. Notice that the name has the "-mycin" ending. Bacteria that have developed resistance to macrolides are often still sensitive to ketolides. Telithromycin also has activity against intracellular respiratory pathogens.

STREPTOGRAMINS AND OXAZOLIDINONES

There are several newer groups of protein synthesis inhibitors. One is the streptogramins. The first drug in this class is the combination of dalfopristin and quinupristin. The two components are always given together because they act synergistically to inhibit ribosome function.

The second group is the oxazolidinones—proudly represented by linezolid and tedizolid. These drugs inhibit protein synthesis by interfering with translation. The predominant activity of linezolid is against aerobic gram-positive organisms and it is approved for vancomycin-resistant infections. It is also an inhibitor of monoamine oxidase. Reduction in MAO activity leads to an increase in the concentration of norepinephrine and can increase blood pressure.

The third group is the pleuromutilins. Retapamulin was the first pleuromutilin available as an antibacterial agent. These drugs interfere with the function of the 50S subunit of the bacterial ribosome. Lefamulin is a newer semisynthetic pleuromutilin that has been approved for the treatment of community acquired pneumonia.

Finally, mupirocin is a topical antibiotic originally isolated from a *Pseudomonas* that inhibits isoleucyl transfer RNA. Be sure to add any other new protein synthesis inhibitors to this section.

CHLORAMPHENICOL

Chloramphenicol is a broad-spectrum antibiotic, effective against most aerobic and anaerobic bacteria, except *Pseudomonas aeruginosa*.

> CHLORAMPHENICOL is associated with bone marrow depression and aplastic anemia that is usually *fatal*.

Chloramphenicol is reserved for life-threatening infections because of its serious, life-threatening adverse effects. A dose-related bone marrow depression can occur, and a dose-related reversible anemia has been reported. An idiosyncratic aplastic anemia (1 in 40,000 cases) can occur that is usually *fatal*.

> CHLORAMPHENICOL can produce gray baby syndrome, which is often *fatal*.

Chloramphenicol is orally absorbed, penetrates the CSF, and is inactivated in the liver by conjugation. Infants have a decreased ability to conjugate chloramphenicol, resulting in high levels in the blood. They develop abdominal distention, vomiting, cyanosis, hypothermia, decreased respiration, and vasomotor collapse.

CLINDAMYCIN

These drugs (clindamycin and lincomycin) are sometimes called lincosamides based on their chemical structure. Notice that they end in "-mycin" but are not related to the aminoglycosides or macrolides. Lincomycin is rarely used, so focus on remembering clindamycin. The antibacterial activity of clindamycin is similar to that of erythromycin.

> Clindamycin penetrates most tissues, including bone. It has activity against anaerobes.

Clindamycin inhibits toxin production, so it is recommended as adjunct therapy when toxin-producing bacteria are suspected. Use of clindamycin is associated with pseudomembranous colitis.

CHAPTER

30

Folate Antagonists

Mechanism of Action
Selected Features

MECHANISM OF ACTION

To understand the mechanism of action of this class of drugs, we need to first review the synthesis of folic acid (Figure 30–1). Bacteria cannot absorb folic acid but must make it from PABA (para-aminobenzoic acid), pteridine, and glutamate. For humans, folic acid is a vitamin. We cannot synthesize it. This makes this metabolic pathway a nice, selective target for antimicrobial agents.

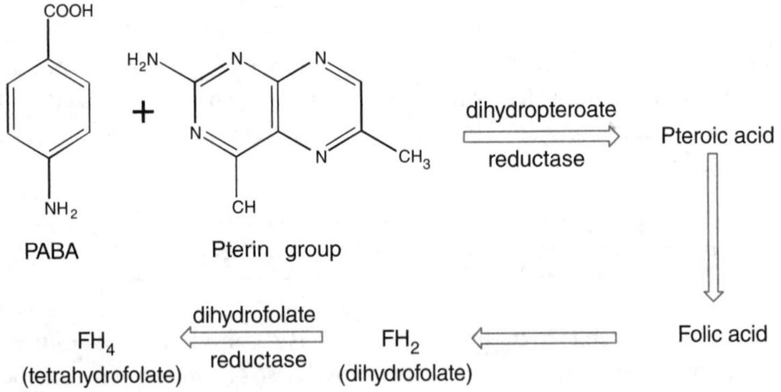

FIGURE 30-1 This figure presents the synthesis of folic acid, for review.

Sulfonamides and trimethoprim inhibit synthesis of folate at two different sites.

The sulfonamides are structurally similar to PABA and block the incorporation of PABA into dihydropteroic acid. Trimethoprim prevents reduction of dihydrofolate to tetrahydrofolate by inhibiting the enzyme dihydrofolate reductase. This enzyme is present in humans, but trimethoprim has a lower affinity for the human enzyme. There are other examples of folate reductase inhibitors that we will consider later (pyrimethamine and methotrexate).

The combination of sulfonamides and trimethoprim is synergistic, and they are rarely used alone. Sulfamethoxazole is the sulfonamide used in combination with trimethoprim because sulfonamides and trimethoprim have matching half-lives.

SULFAMETHOXAZOLE	sulfadiazine
TRIMETHOPRIM	sulfapyridine
cotrimoxazole	sulfasalazine
sulfacetamide	sulfisoxazole

There are other sulfonamides; please check your textbook. Note that sulfasalazine is also used to treat inflammatory bowel disease (see Chapter 44).

SELECTED FEATURES

These folate antagonists are broad-spectrum agents that are effective against gram-positive and gram-negative organisms.

The combination of sulfamethoxazole and trimethoprim, called *cotrimoxazole*, is probably the most commonly used drug in this group. It is used for urinary tract infections and *Pneumocystis carinii* pneumonitis, among other things. These drugs are orally absorbed.

31 Quinolones and Urinary Tract Antiseptics

> Drugs in This Group
> Quinolones
> Methenamine

DRUGS IN THIS GROUP

Quinolones are a group of antimicrobials that were originally used primarily to treat patients with urinary tract infections.

QUINOLONES

- CIPROFLOXACIN
- delafloxacin
- gemifloxacin
- gatifloxacin
- levofloxacin
- ofloxacin
- moxifloxacin
- norfloxacin

For now, the names of the drugs in this class are easy to recognize.

> Quinolones inhibit DNA synthesis through a specific action on DNA gyrase and topoisomerase intravenously (IV).

These drugs inhibit DNA gyrase and, thus, DNA synthesis. DNA gyrase is the bacterial enzyme that is responsible for unwinding and supercoiling of the DNA. This is the only class of antibacterials that inhibits DNA replication. This is a more common approach for the antivirals and the anticancer drugs.

> Quinolones can be used to treat genitourinary, respiratory, gastrointestinal (GI), and some skin and soft tissue infections.

These drugs are considered to be broad-spectrum antimicrobial agents. Nalidixic acid was the first available, and it is an effective urinary tract antiseptic (it sterilizes the urine). The newer agents in this group are useful in a wide range of bacterial infections, including lower respiratory tract infections, bone and joint infections, and prostatitis. Some are effective against *Pseudomonas aeruginosa* and are orally active.

> Quinolones now have a black box warning that they can cause tendinitis, tendon rupture, peripheral neuropathy, and central nervous system (CNS) effects, including delirium, agitation, nervousness and changes in attention, and memory and orientation. A causative link to aortic aneurysm has recently been added to the warning.

Because of the association with serious adverse reactions, clinicians are being warned to reserve these drugs for patients who have no alternative treatment.

METHENAMINE

> Methenamine is metabolized to formaldehyde and ammonia and is used in urinary tract infections.

If you are simply overloaded at this point, skip this drug. Methenamine is an interesting example of a prodrug. The parent compound is not active. In acidic pH, it is hydrolyzed to ammonia and formaldehyde. The formaldehyde is lethal to bacteria. Therefore, this is another bactericidal drug. Methenamine is usually administered as a salt of an acid to help keep the pH of the urine less than 5.5, which is vital for the effective use of methenamine.

32 Drugs Used in Tuberculosis and Leprosy

Organization of Class

Isoniazid

Rifampin

Pyrazinamide

Ethambutol

Dapsone

ORGANIZATION OF CLASS

The mycobacteria that cause tuberculosis and leprosy are very slow growing, so therapy must be continued for relatively long periods of time. The cell wall of these bacteria is more than 60% lipid, mostly mycolic acids. To prevent the emergence of resistant strains, it is vital to employ combination therapy with as many as four or five agents to which the organism is sensitive. The current treatment regimen for tuberculosis (TB) (which is subject to change) is 2 months of isoniazid, rifampin, pyrazinamide, and ethambutol, followed by 4 months of isoniazid and rifampin. Increasing the duration of therapy or changing the choice of drugs depends on culture and sensitivity results and factors that increase risk of treatment failure.

The drugs for TB are most commonly divided into two groups: first-line drugs and second-line drugs. For most purposes, knowledge of the first-line drugs is adequate. If you decide to specialize in infectious disease or the treatment of tuberculosis, a working knowledge of the other drugs is important.

First-Line Drugs	Second-Line Drugs
ISONIAZID	amikacin
PYRAZINAMIDE	aminosalicylic acid
RIFAMPIN	capreomycin
ETHAMBUTOL	cycloserine
	ethionamide

(Continued)

First-Line Drugs	Second-Line Drugs
	kanamycin
	levofloxacin
	moxifloxacin
	rifabutin
	rifapentine
	streptomycin

Streptomycin was covered in more detail in Chapter 29, so we won't consider it again.

ISONIAZID

> ISONIAZID inhibits synthesis of mycolic acids.

Isoniazid is a prodrug that inhibits the synthesis of mycolic acids and nucleic acids.

> There are patients who are fast and slow acetylators of ISONIAZID.

You may have already heard mention of fast and slow acetylators. This is a genetically determined trait. Acetylation is a metabolic pathway for many drugs, but this pathway is of particular importance for isoniazid. Isoniazid has a shorter half-life in fast acetylators.

> ISONIAZID is associated with hepatotoxicity and peripheral neuropathy.

Hepatitis is the most severe side effect of isoniazid. Isoniazid-induced liver dysfunction is reversible, and the incidence increases with age.

The peripheral neuropathy results from pyridoxine deficiency. It can be corrected by pyridoxine (vit B_6) supplementation.

> ISONIAZID is the *drug of choice* for chemoprophylaxis in recent converters.

If a person has had negative TB tests (purified protein derivative [PPD] test) in the past, and then 1 year later the test is positive, that person is said to be a recent converter. The current recommendations (of course, subject to change) is that the person be placed on isoniazid for 9 months, as long as there is no evidence of clinical disease, such as a positive chest x-ray.

RIFAMPIN

> RIFAMPIN inhibits RNA synthesis by formation of a stable complex with the DNA-dependent RNA polymerase.

Rifampin binds to the β subunit of the enzyme, DNA-dependent RNA polymerase. The complex that is formed is inactive, thus blocking RNA synthesis. Resistance to rifampin is caused by a single-step mutation that results in an alteration of the β subunit. Not only is rifampin effective against tuberculosis, but it is also effective against some gram-positive and gram-negative organisms.

> RIFAMPIN is metabolized in the liver and is a potent inducer of the P450 enzymes. It can cause hepatitis and may color secretions a red orange.

Rifampin is deacetylated in the liver to an active metabolite. A drug-induced hepatitis can occur that results in jaundice. In addition, rifampin induces the liver microsomal P450 enzymes. This can lead to increased metabolism of any other drug that is also metabolized by this system.

Rifampin may color urine, feces, saliva, sweat, and tears red-orange. The color can even get into contact lenses.

Rifabutin and rifapentine are analogues of rifampin that have some activity against rifampin-resistant *Mycobacterium tuberculosis*.

PYRAZINAMIDE

> PYRAZINAMIDE is only effective against *M. tuberculosis*. It increases levels of serum uric acid.

Pyrazinamide is an analogue of nicotinamide that is particularly effective against intracellular organisms. Hyperuricemia occurs in all patients, but clinical gout is rare. Pyrazinamide has also been associated with hepatotoxicity.

ETHAMBUTOL

> Ethambutol can cause optic neuritis.

Ethambutol inhibits arabinosyltransferase, an enzyme involved in the assembly of the mycobacterial cell wall. It has an interesting adverse effect that often appears on examinations. Ethambutol can cause optic neuritis, resulting in loss of central vision and impaired red-green discrimination.

DAPSONE

The treatment of leprosy is a very specialized area.

> DAPSONE is the mainstay in the treatment of leprosy. It can cause severe hemolysis in patients deficient in G-6-PD.

For years dapsone was the mainstay of the treatment of patients with leprosy. However, worldwide, the problem of drug resistance is becoming severe. Therefore, current recommendations (again, subject to change) are that all forms of leprosy be treated with a combination of drugs—currently rifampin, clofazimine and dapsone. Dapsone is a structural analogue of PABA and is a competitive inhibitor of folic acid synthesis.

Rifampin is an active antileprosy as well as an anti-TB drug.

33   Antifungal Drugs

Organization of Class
Azole Antifungals
Polyene Antifungals
Echinocandins
Fungal Protein Inhibitors

ORGANIZATION OF CLASS

Fungi are eukaryotes, making it challenging to target the pathogen without significant host toxicity. In addition, many fungal infections occur in poorly vascularized tissues or avascular structures such as the superficial layer of the skin, nails, and hair. Fungi are slow growing and are, therefore, more difficult to kill than bacteria, where cell division can be a target. Because many fungi are opportunistic, host factors play an important role in determining prognosis. The antifungal agents essentially assist the host immune system with the fight against the fungus.

In general, these drugs are poorly soluble and, therefore, distribution to the site of action is often a problem. Consider these issues as you study these drugs. As with the antimicrobials, also consider the issue of host versus invading organism. The drug should attack only the invading (foreign) organism and not the host (human) cells. A common target for antifungals is ergosterol. Ergosterol is a membrane component in fungi that is not found in human cells. Humans use cholesterol. However, compare the structures of ergosterol and cholesterol, and you will find them quite close. This is the basis of many of the adverse effects of these drugs.

Classification can be done in a couple of ways. One of the most obvious ways to classify these drugs is by activity against systemic fungal infections or superficial fungal infections. The systemic infections include diseases such as disseminated blastomycosis or coccidioidomycosis. The superficial mycoses include infections with dermatophytes of the skin, hair, and nails.

A better way to organize the antifungals is by mechanism of action. Then, when new drugs are developed, you have a place to file the information in your brain.

Azoles		
imidazoles (2N)	topical and systemic	triazoles (3N)—systemic
topical	ketoconazole	FLUCONAZOLE
butoconazole	miconazole	isavuconazole
clotrimazole		ITRACONAZOLE
econazole		voriconazole
luliconazole		posaconazole
oxiconazole		terconazole

Polyenes	Others	Echinocandins
AMPHOTERICIN B	flucytosine	anidulafungin
nystatin	griseofulvin	caspofungin
	pentamidine	micafungin
	terbinafine	
	tolnaftate	

AZOLE ANTIFUNGALS

> The azoles are broad-spectrum fungistatic agents that inhibit the synthesis of ergosterol by inhibiting the 14-α-demethylase enzyme.

The azoles are so named because of the nitrogen containing azole ring structure that is part of each of these drugs (Figure 33–1). They are divided into two groups: the imidazoles with two nitrogens in the azole ring, and the triazoles with three nitrogens in the ring. Notice that the names all end in "-azole." This makes recognition of these agents easy.

Compared with the imidazoles, the triazoles tend to have fewer side effects, better drug distribution, and fewer drug interactions. Notice also that the imidazoles are primarily (although not exclusively) topical, whereas the triazoles are active systemically. Different fungal infections have different drugs of choice.

> The azoles antifungals can inhibit cytochrome P450 enzymes. Therefore, this class of drugs is particularly susceptible to clinically significant drug interactions.

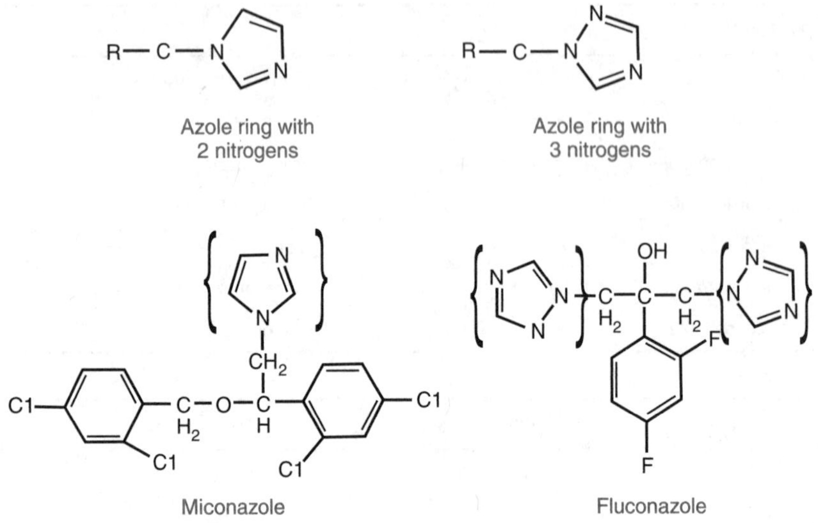

FIGURE 33–1 On the left are the imidazoles with two nitrogens in the azole ring, and on the right are the triazoles with three nitrogens in the azole ring.

POLYENE ANTIFUNGALS

> The polyene antifungals, AMPHOTERICIN B and nystatin, work by forming aggregates with ergosterol, disrupting the membrane structure leading to cell death.

Amphotericin B is the antifungal agent that you should know better than the rest. However, remember that nystatin is also a polyene compound and has the same mechanism of action. Both drugs work by an interaction with ergosterol. Although it is not important to memorize the structures of any of these compounds, do take a moment to look at the structure of amphotericin B in Figure 33–2. Sure looks like a long-chain fatty acid, doesn't it?

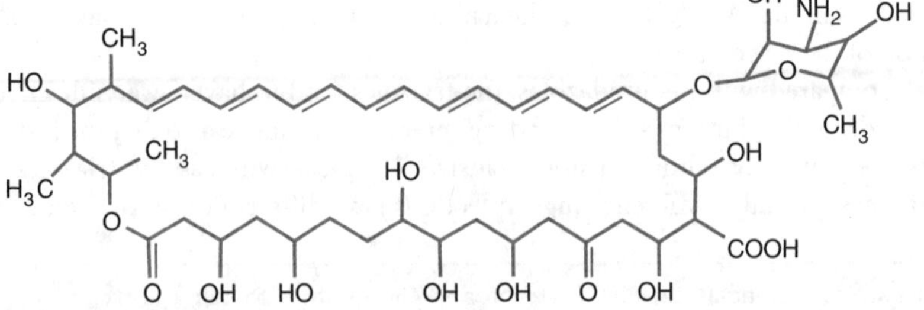

FIGURE 33–2 The structure of amphotericin B is shown here. Doesn't it look an awful lot like a lipid?

> AMPHOTERICIN B is most commonly used to treat serious disseminated yeast and fungal infections, particularly in immunocompromised patients.

Nystatin is too toxic for systemic use. Its use is limited to topical treatment for *Candida albicans*.

> The most serious and most common toxicity of AMPHOTERICIN B is nephrotoxicity.

Nephrotoxicity is related to dose and duration of therapy. Keeping patients well hydrated may reduce the nephrotoxicity. Fever, chills, and tachypnea occur commonly after the initial dose of amphotericin B. Amphotericin is now available in several lipid formulations in an attempt to reduce the toxicity.

> AMPHOTERICIN B is not absorbed from the gastrointestinal (GI) tract, so it must be given intravenously or topically.

ECHINOCANDINS

The echinocandins noncompetitively inhibit the synthesis of a major fungal cell wall component, β-(1,3)-D-glucan, which is not present in mammalian cell walls. Caspofungin, anidulafungin, and micafungin are all active against most *Candida* species and against the mold *Aspergillus*. All three drugs are given intravenously and appear to be similar in safety and efficacy. Note that, for now, the names all end in "-fungin."

FUNGAL PROTEIN INHIBITORS

> Terbinafine prevents ergosterol synthesis by inhibiting squalene epoxidase.

Terbinafine and tolnaftate inhibit squalene epoxidase, resulting in the accumulation of squalene inside the fungal cells. Terbinafine, given orally, is effective against the skin and nail fungi. The target tissues are those that are not well vascularized: hair, skin, and nails. Yet this drug is given orally and not applied topically.

> Tavaborole blocks fungal protein synthesis by inhibiting aminoacyl-transfer ribonucleic acid synthetase.

Careful with the name here. Don't confuse this drug with an azole. Tavaborole is used for onychomycosis (mostly toenails).

> Pentamidine is used to treat *Pneumocystis jiroveci*, which is now classified as a fungus and leishmaniasis and trypanosomiasis, which are protozoa.

Griseofulvin is an older, orally active drug used for dermatophyte infections.

CHAPTER

34

Anthelmintic Drugs

Organization of Class
Drugs Used against Cestodes and Trematodes
Drugs Used against Nematodes
Drugs Used against Filaria

ORGANIZATION OF CLASS

These drugs are effective against worms (helminths). In humans, worms may remain within the intestinal lumen or may have complex life cycles that involve movement through the body. The infective form may be either an adult worm or an immature worm.

The worm life cycle is strongly dependent on neuromuscular coordination, energy production, and microtubular integrity. Most antiworm drugs target one of these three areas.

The easiest way to organize these drugs is to consider a reasonable organization of the worms. Helminths (worms) are classified into three groups: cestodes (flatworms), nematodes (roundworms), and trematodes (flukes). If you look at the table of worms and the drug of choice for each worm, several patterns emerge.

Helminth	Drug of Choice
Cestodes (flatworms and tapeworms)	ALBENDAZOLE/MEBENDAZOLE
	PRAZIQUANTEL
Trematodes (flukes [schistosomiasis])	PRAZIQUANTEL, triclabendazole
Nematodes (ascaris, pinworm, hookworm)	ALBENDAZOLE/MEBENDAZOLE
	PYRANTEL
Filariasis	ivermectin/diethylcarbamazine

DRUGS USED AGAINST CESTODES AND TREMATODES

PRAZIQUANTEL is the *drug of choice* for most trematode (flukes) and many cestode infections.

First, here's a quick review of the worms. Cestodes are the tapeworms. They are flat and segmented. The head has suckers. Larvae develop into adults in the small intestine. Therefore, treatment can be confined to the small intestine.

The trematodes are the flukes. If you recall, the flukes move about the body; there are blood flukes and liver flukes, and so on. Therefore, the treatment needs to reach the systemic circulation in order to affect the fluke.

The mechanism of action of praziquantel is unknown. It is postulated to alter membrane function of the worm and increase membrane permeability. It is absorbed after oral administration. That's why it can have an action on the trematodes (flukes) that cause schistosomiasis.

DRUGS USED AGAINST NEMATODES

Treatment of nematodes (roundworms) consists of (for the most part) ALBENDAZOLE, MEBENDAZOLE, or PYRANTEL.

The nematodes are a more diverse set of worms. Overall, they are the roundworms because they are elongated and cylindrical (round). This group includes whipworm, pinworm, and hookworm. In the United States, the most common helminth infections are ascaris lumbricoides, ancylostoma duodenale (roundworm), and necator americanus (hookworm). Most patients with nematode infections can be treated using mebendazole or pyrantel. A special group of nematodes can be considered separately: the filaria. Patients with filariasis are treated using two other drugs.

ALBENDAZOLE and MEBENDAZOLE inhibit tubulin polymerization in the worms.

These drugs bind to β-tubulin and inhibit tubulin polymerization, which disrupts motility and replication. They can be given orally, and very little is absorbed from the gastrointestinal (GI) tract.

PYRANTEL causes paralysis of the worms.

DRUGS USED AGAINST FILARIA

Filariasis is treated (for the most part) with ivermectin or diethylcarbamazine.

Filaria are threadlike worms that are found in blood and tissue. They are transmitted by the bite of a fly or mosquito. Early in the infection, they move through the lymphatic system.

Diethylcarbamazine is the *drug of choice* for lymphatic filariasis.

Diethylcarbamazine is not commercially available in the United States but can be obtained from the Centers for Disease Control and Prevention (CDC). This drug appears to alter the surface of the filaria in such a way that they are more susceptible to phagocytosis by the host immune system.

> Ivermectin paralyzes the worm muscle and is the *drug of choice* for onchocerciasis (river blindness).

Ivermectin is more commonly known in veterinary medicine but has found a niche in the treatment of onchocerciasis. It appears to block γ-aminobutyric acid (GABA)–mediated transmission in the invading organism without any effect on the host. Elimination of onchocerciasis worldwide has been hampered by coinfections with *Loa loa*. Patients with *Loa loa* can develop serious adverse effects after treatment with ivermectin.

Antiviral Drugs

Organization of Class
Anti-HIV Drugs
Drugs Used in Influenza (RNA virus)
Drugs Used in Hepatitis B and C
Other Antivirals

ORGANIZATION OF CLASS

Three basic approaches are taken to control viral diseases. Vaccination is used to try to prevent and control the spread of disease. Chemotherapy (the focus of pharmacology) is used to treat the symptoms of viral illness and to try to eliminate the virus from the body. Finally, stimulation of the host's natural resistance mechanisms is used to shorten the duration of illness.

The problems with chemotherapy are similar to those discussed for antimicrobial and antifungal agents. Anytime we are trying to kill an invading (foreign) organism, there is the problem of the drug recognizing and distinguishing the invading organism from the host. To understand the antiviral agents, it is necessary to review the life cycle of viruses and imagine sites where drugs could interfere or block:

1. Attachment and penetration of the virus to the host cell.
2. Uncoating of the viral genome within the host cell.
3. Synthesis of viral components within the host cell.
4. Assembly of viral particles.
5. Release of the virus to spread and invade other cells.

Most of the drugs that are currently available block specific viral proteins that are involved in synthesis of viral components within the host cell.

ANTI-HIV DRUGS

Reverse Transcriptase Inhibitors			Protease Inhibitors	Fusion and Entry Inhibitors
NRTIs	**NNRTIs**	**nucleotide**	atazanavir	enfuvirtide
abacavir	delavirdine	tenofovir	darunavir	maraviroc
didanosine	doravirine		fosamprenavir	
emtricitabine	efavirenz		indinavir	**Integrase Inhibitors**
lamivudine	etravirine		lopinavir	bictegravir
stavudine	nevirapine		nelfinavir	dolutegravir
zidovudine	rilpivirine		ritonavir	elvitegravir
			saquinavir	raltegravir
			tipranavir	

As a reminder, human immunodeficiency virus (HIV), which is the virus that causes AIDS, is an RNA retrovirus. This means that it has a specific enzyme called *reverse transcriptase*. This is a major target of drugs with efficacy against HIV.

> The nucleoside (NRTIs), nucleotide, and nonnucleoside (NNRTIs) reverse transcriptase inhibitors (RT inhibitors) all inhibit the formation of viral DNA from RNA by reverse transcriptase.

The RT inhibitors are divided into several groups based on whether they are structurally related to nucleoside/nucleotides or not. The nucleoside analogues are related to thymidine and adenosine and, after triple phosphorylation, are incorporated into viral DNA during the reverse transcription of the viral RNA. But because they are not exactly the same as the native nucleosides, there is early termination of DNA elongation. The nucleotide RT inhibitor works in a similar manner, except that it is already phosphorylated once. The nonnucleoside inhibitors also stop the reverse transcriptase enzyme, but not by mimicking the natural nucleosides.

Mutation of the reverse transcriptase enzyme is very rapid. The use of at least two RT inhibitors simultaneously slows the emergence of resistant virus.

> The protease inhibitors interfere with processing of the viral protein, thus preventing formation of new viral particles.

The HIV protease enzyme is involved in maturation of the newly formed viral particle. These drugs have a number of side effects, including changes in fat deposition and metabolic abnormalities.

> It is now common practice to combine protease inhibitors with a low dose of ritonavir or cobicistat because these drugs inhibit CYP3A4 metabolism.

Cobicistat is a ritonavir analogue that lacks antiretroviral activity and is used exclusively as a "kinetic enhancer." It is better tolerated than ritonavir and inhibits both first-pass metabolism and systemic clearance. This allows a reduction in drug dose and dosing frequency.

> Enfuvirtide blocks the fusion of the viral particle to the target cell, while maraviroc inhibits entry of the viral particles into cells.

Enfuvirtide is an analogue of the HIV protein that mediates fusion with the cell membrane. When enfuvirtide binds in place of the HIV protein, it traps the viral particle in a conformation that prevents its fusion with the cell—thus the term *fusion inhibitor*. Enfuvirtide has to be given by injection. Maraviroc blocks one of the proteins (CCR5) that acts as a receptor for the HIV virus. Maraviroc is only active against HIV strains that are "R5 tropic."

> Integrase inhibitors, used in combination, are first-line drugs for newly diagnosed HIV patients.

One key feature of HIV infection is that the virus integrates itself into the host cells genome, thus becoming part of the cell. This is mediated by a viral enzyme called *integrase*. Blocking this enzyme could potentially keep cells from becoming permanently infected with the HIV virus.

> Therapy for HIV is based on combinations of drugs that provide multiple mechanisms of action and reduced side effects.

Current recommendations for drug treatment can be found at www.aidsinfo.nih.gov.

DRUGS USED IN INFLUENZA (RNA VIRUS)

The mainstay of protection against influenza has always been vaccination. Drugs are now available that effectively treat influenza if started early in the infection.

Influenza Drugs	Neuraminidase Inhibitors	CAP Endonuclease inhibitor
AMANTADINE	oseltamivir	baloxavir
rimantadine	peramivir	
	zanamivir	

> AMANTADINE is used for the prevention and treatment of influenza type A infections.

If begun within 48 hours of the onset of illness, amantadine shortens the duration of symptoms by about half. The use of amantadine is limited by rapid emergence of resistance and by the drug's adverse effects.

> Neuraminidase inhibitors block release of influenza virus from infected cells.

The neuraminidase inhibitors work by inhibiting an enzyme located on the surface of the virus that breaks a bond between the virus and proteins on the cell surface, thus allowing formed viral particles to be released. The active site of the neuraminidase enzyme is a highly conserved site in both types A and B influenza. The neuraminidase inhibitors bind to the active site and block it. Use of these agents is reported to shorten the duration of symptomatic illness if the drug is started within 30 hours of the onset of symptoms.

Baloxavir marboxil is synergistic with the neuraminidase inhibitors. It inhibits a subdomain of the viral RNA polymerase called *CAP endonuclease*. Baloxavir has been found to shorten the duration of symptoms.

DRUGS USED IN HEPATITIS B AND C

There are five main hepatitis viruses (A, B, C, D, and E). Vaccines are available for all, EXCEPT hepatitis C. Hepatitis A and E are spread by lack of food hygiene, contaminated water, and substandard sanitary facilities. Hepatitis B, C, and D are spread by blood, serum, and other bodily fluids. Hepatitis A and E are typically self-limiting, and there are no antiviral therapies for them. Hepatitis B and C can progress to chronic infection putting patients at risk for cirrhosis, liver failure, and hepatocellular carcinoma. Hepatitis C is the leading indication for liver transplantation.

Hepatitis B (dsDNA)	Hepatitis C (ssRNA)	
adefovir	NS5A inhibitors	NS5B inhibitors
entecavir	daclatasvir	dasabuvir
interferon-α (first-line)	elbasvir	sofosbuvir
lamivudine	ledipasvir	NS3/4A protease inhibitors
telbivudine	ombitasvir	glecaprevir
tenofovir	pibrentasvir	grazoprevir
	velpatasvir	paritaprevir
		meprevir
		Other
		ritonavir—booster

Notice that some of the drugs listed for hepatitis B are also on the list for the treatment of HIV. Chronic hepatitis B is currently treated with weekly injections with interferon-α or daily oral treatment with a nucleoside/nucleotide analogue such as lamivudine or telbivudine over long periods of time.

First, notice that all of the drugs for hepatitis C end in "vir," as do many of the HIV drugs. At least, you should recognize them as antiviral agents.

There are six distinct genotypes of hepatitis C virus, and there are differing recommendations based on the genotype of the infection. However, learning that level of specificity at this time is too much. The virus has several proteins that are targets of drug therapy. NS5A is a viral protein essential for replication and new virus assembly. NS3/4A protease is involved in cleavage of the viral polyprotein. NS5b is an RNA-dependent RNA polymerase. The hepatitis C drugs are used in combination. Again, we see that targeting specific pathways or specific viral proteins is an effective way to develop treatment options. Treatment of hepatitis C is a rapidly evolving field, and you should get the latest on testing and treating hepatitis C online.

OTHER ANTIVIRALS

Other Antivirals	
Herpes (DNA)	**RSV**
ACYCLOVIR (valacyclovir)	RIBAVIRIN
ganciclovir (valganciclovir)	palivizumab
penciclovir (famciclovir)	
vidarabine (ara-A)	
cidofovir	

Herpes simplex virus type I typically causes disease of the mouth, face, skin, esophagus, or brain. HSV-2 usually causes infections of the genitals, rectum, skin, or meninges. Drugs used to treat herpes infections do so by inhibiting viral DNA replication.

ACYCLOVIR is used to treat patients with herpes infections. To be effective, it must be activated by triple phosphorylation.

Acyclovir is used topically, intravenously, and orally for the treatment of patients with herpes infections. Valacyclovir is a prodrug of acyclovir with better bioavailability. As with the anti-HIV nucleoside RT inhibitors, acyclovir must undergo a triple phosphorylation to an active derivative. Acyclovir triphosphate inhibits the herpes virus DNA polymerase. A number of other "-ciclovir" drugs are also used against herpes infections.

Ganciclovir or valganciclovir (prodrug) is the best choice for infections with cytomegalovirus.

RIBAVIRIN is used in the treatment of respiratory syncytial virus (RSV) in infants and young children.

The mechanism of action of ribavirin is unknown, but it is felt to be an antimetabolite. It is used in aerosol form for the treatment of RSV in young children. This could be labeled as a *drug of choice*. Palivizumab is a humanized monoclonal antibody against a glycoprotein on the surface of the virus. It is given as an injection at the start of RSV season in high-risk children to provide passive immunity.

Note about coronaviruses. To date (early 2021) there are no specific treatments for any of the infections caused by coronaviruses. Remdesivir is a nucleotide prodrug of an adenosine analogue that inhibits viral RNA polymerase. It is active against a variety of coronaviruses. Emergency use authorization has been given to a couple of monoclonal antibodies that bind to the spike protein of SARS-CoV-2—bamlanivimab and etesevimab. They are to be given together for treatment of mild to moderate COVID-19 in patients at high risk for disease progression.

Antiprotozoal Drugs

Organization of Class
Metronidazole
Antimalarial Agents
Therapeutic Considerations
Special Features

ORGANIZATION OF CLASS

To simplify the discussion, the antimalarial drugs are covered in a separate section at the end of this chapter. Some of the more common protozoal diseases are listed in the following table.

Protozoa	Disease
Entamoeba histolytica	Amebiasis (diarrhea)
Balantidium coli	Balantidial dysentery
Trichomonas vaginalis	Trichomoniasis (genital infection)
Giardia lamblia	Giardiasis (diarrhea)
Leishmania	Leishmaniasis (three types)
Trypanosoma brucei	African sleeping sickness
Trypanosoma cruzi	Chagas disease (South American)

Of the drugs used in these diseases, metronidazole is most important for you to know. Of the diseases listed, trichomoniasis and giardiasis are most common in the United States and both are treated with metronidazole. This along with a few more details will go a long way. You need to be aware of the other drugs and where to find the information about treatment for these diseases.

Antiprotozoal Drugs	
METRONIDAZOLE	nifurtimox (Chagas)
benznidazole (Chagas)	pentamidine (African sleeping sickness)
eflornithine (African sleeping sickness)	sodium stibogluconate (leishmaniasis)
miltefosine (leishmaniasis)	suramin (African sleeping sickness)
nitazoxanide (cryptosporidiosis)	tinidazole

METRONIDAZOLE

> METRONIDAZOLE is effective in the treatment of vaginal trichomoniasis, giardiasis, and all forms of amebiasis.

First note that metronidazole, fenbendazole, and tinidazole end in "azole" but are not antifungal agents. Sorry!

Metronidazole is one of the most effective drugs against anaerobic bacteria and several protozoal species. It is highly effective in the treatment of trichomoniasis. It penetrates protozoal and bacterial cell walls but cannot enter mammalian cells. The drug must be activated once it has entered the cell. The activating enzyme, nitroreductase, is found only in anaerobic organisms. The reduced metronidazole inhibits DNA replication by causing breaks and inhibiting repair of the DNA.

The most common side effects are nausea, vomiting, and diarrhea. The drug can turn the urine dark or red-brown and cause a metallic taste in the mouth. Metronidazole can cause a disulfiram-like reaction when taken with alcohol. The disulfiram-like effect consists of abdominal cramping, vomiting, flushing, or headache after drinking alcohol.

ANTIMALARIAL AGENTS

Malaria is caused by a single-cell protozoa, the plasmodium. There are over 50 species of plasmodia, but only 4 are infectious to humans: *Plasmodium malariae*, *Plasmodium ovale*, *Plasmodium vivax*, and *Plasmodium falciparum*. *Plasmodium vivax* is the most prevalent, but *P. falciparum* is the most serious and lethal form of malaria.

To understand the drugs and the rationale behind treatment of patients with malaria, it is important to understand the life cycle of the malaria organism (Figure 36–1).

Notice that only *P. vivax* and *P. ovale* can persist in the liver and, therefore, patients infected with these species can relapse.

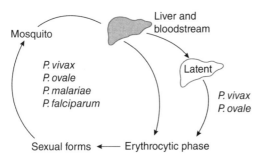

FIGURE 36-1 As a reminder, the life cycle of the malaria-causing protozoa is presented. *Plasmodium vivax* and *Plasmodium ovale* are the two species that can take up residence in the liver.

THERAPEUTIC CONSIDERATIONS

It is thought that the symptoms are caused by the erythrocytic form of the parasite. Therefore, elimination of this asexual form will relieve symptoms. Drugs that do this are called *suppressive* or *schizonticidal* agents.

The emergence of chloroquine-resistant organisms is becoming a major health concern. The nuances of treatment of resistant organisms will not be addressed here, but you can find current treatment strategies at the Centers for Disease Control and Prevention (CDC) website.

ANTI-MALARIAL DRUGS	
artemisinins	hydroxychloroquine
CHLOROQUINE	mefloquine
PRIMAQUINE/tafenoquine	pyrimethamine
QUININE	tafenoquine
doxycycline	

To treat all strains, except those resistant to chloroquine, chloroquine is the oral drug of choice. That should be easy to remember. For parenteral use, quinidine and quinine are the drugs of choice. However, resistance is a major problem worldwide.

> ARTEMETHER-LUMEFANTRINE is highly effective for the treatment of uncomplicated malaria, including multidrug resistant infections.

Artemisinins are Chinese herbal products that have been shown to be quite effective against malaria. The active components are artemether and artesunate. Artemether inhibits nucleic acid and protein biosynthesis and is approved in the United States in combination with lumefantrine.

SPECIAL FEATURES

> PRIMAQUINE is effective against liver forms (exoerythrocytic) and kills gametocytes.

Because of its effectiveness against the liver phases, primaquine is often used for prophylaxis or prevention of relapse.

> PRIMAQUINE can cause hemolytic anemia in glucose-6-phosphate dehydrogenase (G6PD)–deficient patients.

Do you remember the G6PD enzyme? In biochemistry, you probably learned that some people are deficient in this enzyme and should avoid taking certain drugs. Primaquine is one of those drugs. This is an important (albeit somewhat specific) fact.

Chloroquine, in low doses, is not very toxic. However, in high doses or for long durations of treatment, it can cause toxicity of the skin, blood, and eyes. (Note: This is different from the standard nausea, vomiting, and diarrhea.) The drug becomes concentrated in melanin-containing structures, and this can lead to corneal deposits and blindness.

The mechanism of action of quinine is unknown. Quinine is derived from the bark of the cinchona tree, and the name given to describe quinine toxicity—cinchonism—reflects this. Cinchonism consists of sweating, ringing in the ears, impaired hearing, blurred vision, and nausea, vomiting, and diarrhea.

Chloroquine is also used for prophylaxis for travelers entering areas where chloroquine-sensitive malaria is endemic.

Anticancer Drugs

Organization of Class
Terminology and General Principles of Therapy
Adverse Effects
Cytotoxic Drugs
    Alkylating Agents
    Antimetabolites
    Antibiotics and Other Natural Products
    Other Cytotoxic Drugs
Hormonal Agents
Pathway-targeted Therapies
    Growth Factors and Receptors
    Intracellular Kinases
    Angiogenesis
    Other Targets
Miscellaneous Agents

ORGANIZATION OF CLASS

The anticancer drugs usually follow the antimicrobials in most pharmacology textbooks. This is because the drugs, in many cases, are similar.

Many students get really bogged down with the anticancer drugs. There are an awful lot of drugs with known mechanisms of action and multiple side effects that can be quite serious. However, there are some general principles of the use of these drugs that can be emphasized. In fact, these principles are more important than the individual agents. So, for the purposes of this book, focus on name recognition (be sure that you recognize a particular agent as an anticancer drug) and a few specific toxicities. Do not try to remember every type of cancer that the drug is used for. You can add some of this information later as you use these drugs in the clinical setting. Get a handle on the overall picture before you focus on the details.

Another annoying thing about this group of drugs is that some of these agents are known by several names.

> *Cytotoxic drugs—drugs which block cell replication*
>
> Alkylating agents, including nitrogen mustards and nitrosoureas
> Antimetabolites, including folate antagonists, purine and pyrimidine analogues
> Antibiotics and other natural products, including anthracyclines and vinca alkaloids
> Other cytotoxic drugs
>
> *Hormonal agents—drugs for hormone-sensitive tumors*
> *Pathway-targeted therapy*

The drugs can be divided into three simple groups: the cytotoxic drugs, hormones, and pathway-targeted therapies. All of the alkylating agents, antibiotics, antimetabolites, and miscellaneous drugs are cytotoxic drugs—they kill cells, particularly dividing cells. Therefore, all of the following terminology and general principles apply to the cytotoxic drugs. The hormonal agents are used for tumors of the hormonally sensitive tissues, such as breast and prostate. As always there are some drugs that do not fit neatly into these two categories.

TERMINOLOGY AND GENERAL PRINCIPLES OF THERAPY

> Anticancer therapy is aimed at killing dividing cells. There are normal host cells that are also dividing. Effects on these cells cause side effects.

This is a bit simplistic but serves our purposes for now. In antimicrobial therapy, the object is to kill the invading bacteria without harming the host. In anticancer therapy, the object is to kill the cancer cells without harming the normal cells. This is difficult because the cancer cells are also human (or host) cells. The cancer cells are basically human cells that have lost control of cell division. Therefore, anticancer treatment is, in large part, aimed at killing dividing cells. Remember that cells in certain places in the body—the epithelium of the gastrointestinal (GI) tract, hair follicles, and bone marrow, especially—are dividing continuously. Effects on these dividing cells cause adverse effects.

Because many of these drugs target dividing cells, the cell cycle is important to remember (Figure 37–1). When known, textbooks will list the part of the cell cycle in which a drug has an effect or they will list that a drug is cell cycle specific or not. This is not critical information for your first pass through the material. However, as you learn more about the tumors and their growth rates, this information should be added.

The anticancer drugs act by first-order kinetics. Remember kinetics? This means that a constant fraction of the cells (say, 50%) are killed by one dose. This is quite different from a constant number of cells being killed. If one dose of the drug kills 50% of the tumor cells, a second dose of the drug will kill 50% of the remaining tumor cells. This results in a 75% reduction in the number of tumor cells after two doses of this drug. The number of tumor cells is usually expressed in exponentials.

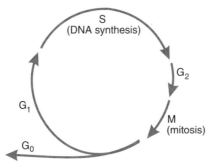

FIGURE 37-1 Cells go through several cycles around cell division. DNA synthesis occurs during the S phase and the actual division takes place during the M phase.

> The log kill is an important concept to understand. The anticancer drugs kill a constant fraction of cells instead of an absolute number.

This is why the so-called kill of a drug is described in log units. The drug that reduces the tumor cell load from 10^8 to 10^5 cells is said to have achieved a "3 log kill."

> Drug resistance to anticancer drugs is analogous to resistance to antimicrobials.

Cancer cells already contain a mutation that allows unrestricted growth. They can also mutate in a way that makes them resistant to anticancer drugs.

> Combinations of drugs are frequently used in the treatment of cancer.

Combinations of drugs reduce the incidence of drug resistance. In addition, the drugs used together often target different phases of the cell cycle or one of the drugs is non–cell cycle specific. The common drug combinations often have acronyms, such as MOPP, VAMP, or POMP, which stand for the individual drugs in the combination. It is not necessary at this time to learn the drug combinations.

ADVERSE EFFECTS

As previously mentioned, the adverse effects of these drugs result from their effects on proliferating cells in the body. We will consider the toxicity of these drugs separately because the principles behind the toxicity are more important than remembering which drugs have more, or less, of a particular toxicity.

> Bone marrow toxicity is caused by destruction of proliferating hematopoietic stem cells. This results in a decrease in all blood elements, including white cells and platelets.

Patients receiving anticancer drugs are at increased risk of developing life-threatening infections and bleeding. This is due to the decrease in white blood cells and platelets. Growth factors are now available that can be used to stimulate cell production in the bone marrow. Fil*grastim* (*granulocyte colony-stim*ulating factor) is used to accelerate recovery of neutrophils and sar*gramostim* (granulocyte-macrophage colony-*stim*ulating factor) is used to accelerate bone marrow repopulation after chemotherapy, radiation, and bone marrow transplantation. Thrombopoietin and erythropoietin can be used to stimulate formation of platelets and red blood cells, respectively. Plerixafor, a CXCR4 chemokine receptor antagonist, can be used in combination with granulocyte colony-stimulating factor to mobilize peripheral stem cells.

> Gastrointestinal (GI) toxicity takes two forms. First, nausea and vomiting due to an effect in the central nervous system (CNS). Second, direct damage to the proliferating mucosa of the GI tract.

Almost all of the cancer chemotherapy drugs cause nausea and vomiting (of course, some are worse than others). It is felt that the drugs stimulate the chemoreceptor trigger zone in the brain that leads to vomiting. Serotonin antagonists (specifically 5-HT$_3$), such as ONDANSETRON, dolasetron, granisetron, and palonosetron, have proven effective in the prevention of nausea and vomiting. (Notice that they all end in "-setron.") A different type of antiemetic are the substance P neurokinin-1 receptor antagonists—aprepitant, netupitant (used in combination with palonosetron), and rolapitant (notice the common endings). Neurokinin-1 receptors are present in the emesis center in the medulla. Protection against vomiting can be enhanced by using both 5-HT$_3$ and neurokinin-1 antagonists in combination with a glucocorticoid. Synthetic cannabinoids (dronabinol and nabilone) are also available for the treatment of chemotherapy-induced nausea and vomiting.

The more predictable effect of the anticancer drugs is killing the proliferating cells in the mucosa of the GI tract. Remember that the epithelium of the GI tract is constantly replicating. These drugs kill dividing cells. Therefore, they will damage the epithelium of the GI tract. This can lead to ulcer formation anywhere in the GI tract—mouth, esophagus, stomach, and so on.

> Most anticancer drugs damage hair follicles and produce hair loss.

This is especially true with cyclophosphamide, doxorubicin, vincristine, methotrexate, and dactinomycin. (Do not worry too much about this for now.)

> Renal tubular damage is the major side effect of cisplatin and high-dose methotrexate. Cyclophosphamide can cause hemorrhagic cystitis.

Renal damage is not that common after use of the anticancer drugs. However, it is a significant side effect of a few drugs. So, learn these few. For many of the drugs, adequate hydration is recommended. But details like these should be added later. MESNA is used to prevent the hemorrhagic cystitis after cyclophosphamide.

> Cardiotoxicity is associated with the use of doxorubicin and daunorubicin (the anthracyclines).

Cardiotoxicity is relatively rare with the anticancer drugs. However, there are two drugs that stand out in this category—the two "D-rubicins." This particular adverse effect has a habit of showing up on board examinations and other such places. Dexrazoxane is a cardioprotective iron-chelating agent used with the anthracyclines.

> Bleomycin can cause pulmonary fibrosis, which can be *fatal*.

This is another example of a particular drug-adverse effect pair that has a habit of showing up in predictable locations, such as exams. It's not too hard to memorize.

> Vincristine is known for its nervous system toxicity.

Vincristine is the only anticancer drug that has a dose-limiting neurotoxicity. Anytime we can use the word *only*, you should try to remember it.

CYTOTOXIC DRUGS

ALKYLATING AGENTS

> Alkylating agents all work by adding an alkyl group to DNA.

These drugs all form highly reactive ion intermediates that covalently link to sites on DNA, thus interfering with DNA integrity and function. These drugs are not cycle specific. They are prone to cause local tissue necrosis and damage.

A. *Nitrogen mustards*	C. *Other alkylating agents*
bendamustine	busulphan
chlorambucil	carboplatin
cyclophosphamide	cisplatin
ifosfamide	oxaliplatin
mechlorethamine (nitrogen mustard)	dacarbazine
melphalan	temozolomide
B. *Nitrosoureas*	thiotepa
carmustine	
lomustine	

The nitrosoureas are easy to recognize because of the "-mustine" ending on their names. They are lipid soluble and therefore cross into the central nervous system (CNS). They have found use in the treatment of brain tumors.

The other alkylating agents—well, if you can remember the names—great.

ANTIMETABOLITES

The antimetabolites compete for binding sites on enzymes or can be incorporated into DNA or RNA. They are especially useful if they bind to an enzyme that has a major effect on pathways leading to cell replication. That should make sense.

> Methotrexate competitively inhibits dihydrofolate reductase.

Remember this pathway from the discussion of folate antagonists? (See Figure 30–1.) Well, methotrexate inhibits DNA synthesis by inhibiting thymidylate synthesis. Cellular uptake of methotrexate is by a carrier-mediated active transport. Cellular resistance to methotrexate is presumably caused by decreased transport into the cell. This can be overcome by using high doses.

There are newer drugs related to methotrexate—pralatrexate, raltitrexed, lometrexol, and pemetrexed.

> Leucovorin provides reduced folate to "rescue" normal cells from the action of methotrexate.

Even before you took pharmacology, you had probably heard of leucovorin rescue during cancer treatment. Leucovorin provides cells with reduced folate, thus bypassing the blocked enzyme.

The other drugs in this group mimic purines or pyrimidines. They get incorporated into the growing DNA during cell division and block further DNA replication. Thus, they are most effective in dividing cells.

A. Purine analogues	B. Pyrimidine analogues
cladribine	capecitabine (prodrug for 5-FU)
fludarabine	cytarabine (cytosine arabinoside, ara-C)
mercaptopurine (6-mercaptopurine)	fluorouracil (5-FU)
pentostatin	gemcitabine
thioguanine (6-thioguanine)	

> The purine and pyrimidine analogues all have to be activated (phosphorylated) before they are effective.

Compare this activation to that of the antivirals (see Chapter 35). Similarities are good—make the mechanisms easier to remember.

ANTIBIOTICS AND OTHER NATURAL PRODUCTS

A. *Anthracyclines*	C. *Vinca alkaloids*
daunorubicin (daunomycin)	vinblastine
doxorubicin	vincristine
epirubicin	vinorelbine
idarubicin	D. *Other natural products*
B. *Other antibiotics*	camptothecin
bleomycin	docetaxel, cabazitaxel
dactinomycin (actinomycin D)	paclitaxel
mitomycin (mitomycin C)	etoposide
plicamycin (mithramycin)	topotecan
	irinotecan

As you can see, there are an awful lot of drugs. Notice that under the antibiotics and natural products, there are a number of drugs that end in "-mycin." Be careful not to confuse these with the anti-microbials that have the same ending.

> The antibiotics all disrupt DNA function.

Most of these drugs bind in some way to DNA. It is easiest to divide the antibiotics into two groups: the anthracyclines and the others.

> The anthracyclines have cardiac toxicity.

The anthracyclines are so named because of their structure. However, the structure is not of primary importance to us. The cardiac toxicity is the most important thing to know about the "-rubicins." Highlight it, make a flash card, do whatever it takes to get you to remember this. The cardiac problems include arrhythmias, decreased function, myofibrillar degeneration, and focal necrosis of myocytes. It is felt that clinical cardiac damage occurs with each dose. It has been postulated that the damage is caused by free radical generation and lipid peroxidation. There is a drug available to help protect the cardiac muscle from this anthracycline-induced toxicity—dexrazoxane. Dexrazoxane chelates intracellular iron. Then the iron cannot react with superoxide anions and hydrogen peroxide to produce the highly toxic-free radicals.

Now on to the other antibiotics, the "-mycins."

> Bleomycin can cause *fatal* pulmonary fibrosis. It does not have significant myelosuppressive effects.

> Plicamycin (mithramycin) can be used to treat life-threatening hypercalcemia associated with malignancy.

Plicamycin inhibits resorption of bone by osteoblasts, thus lowering serum calcium. This fact also appears in the oddest of places.

Let's move on to the other plant products, or naturally occurring agents.

> The vinca alkaloids (vincristine, vinblastine, and vinorelbine) bind to tubulin and disrupt the spindle apparatus during cell division.

These three drugs are the most important ones for you to know.

> For vincristine, the neurological toxicity is dose-limiting. For vinblastine and vinorelbine, the bone marrow toxicity is dose-limiting.

If you can remember that one has neurological toxicity and the other two have bone marrow toxicity, then notice that vinblastine and vinorelbine (the ones with the "b" in the name) are bone marrow toxic.

> Paclitaxel works by preventing depolymerization of microtubules.

Paclitaxel is isolated from the rare Pacific yew tree and quantities are very limited. Docetaxel and cabazitaxel are semisynthetic. Ixabepilone is a semisynthetic drug that also binds to microtubules, so while it's not included in the list of natural products, it deserves a mention here.

> Camptothecin and analogues (topotecan and irinotecan) inhibit topoisomerase I, a nuclear enzyme that allows DNA to replicate.

These three drugs are further down on the trivia list. Learn the names if you have time and energy. They are noted here so that you do not generalize the tubulin action to all the natural plant products.

OTHER CYTOTOXIC DRUGS

asparaginase

hydroxyurea

mitotane

mitoxantrone

procarbazine (*N*-methyl-hydrazine, alkylating)

There are numerous other anticancer drugs. Some of these are occasionally classi-fied as alkylating agents (procarbazine). Please compare the earlier listing to that in your textbook or class handouts.

Hydroxyurea inhibits ribonucleotide reductase.

Mitotane is used to treat adrenocortical adenocarcinoma.

HORMONAL AGENTS

A. *Glucocorticoids*

B. *Aromatase inhibitors*

anastrozole

exemestane

formestane

letrozole

C. *Estrogens/antiestrogens*

fulvestrant (antagonist)

tamoxifen (SERM)

toremifene (SERM)

D. *Androgen receptor antagonists*

bicalutamide

enzalutamide/apalutamide/darolutamide (block signaling)

flutamide

nilutamide

E. *GnRH analogues and antagonists*

abarelix (antagonist)

degarelix (antagonist)

goserelin (analogue)

leuprolide (antagonist/analogue)

triptorelin (analogue)

F. *Inhibit androgen synthesis*

abiraterone

ketoconazole

These drugs are used to treat hormonally sensitive tumors, such as tumors of the breast, prostate, and uterus. The side effects of the drugs are related to the hormonal changes that they induce and not to cytotoxic actions. The goal is to (1) reduce the levels of the hormone that is stimulating growth of the tumor or (2) block the receptor for the hormone.

> Aromatase inhibitors block estrogen formation and are used to treat estrogen-dependent tumors (breast cancer) resistant to tamoxifen.

Estrogen is synthesized from androgen precursors by an enzyme called aromatase. Therefore, inhibiting this enzyme will reduce the production of estrogen. Anastrozole and letrozole are competitive inhibitors of aromatase. Notice that they are *not* "azoles," which are antifungal drugs, but they are both "ozoles." Exemestane (irreversible) and formestane (the "mestanes") bind covalently to the enzyme.

> Tamoxifen and toremifene are competitive antagonists of the estrogen receptor, used in the treatment of breast cancer.

In addition to the competitive antagonists of the estrogen receptor, fulvestrant also works as an estrogen-receptor antagonist. However, in contrast to tamoxifen it downregulates the estrogen receptor.

> The "lutamides" are competitive testosterone antagonists that are used to treat prostate cancer.

> Both GnRH analogues and antagonists will decrease serum levels of estrogen and testosterone and are used to treat androgen-dependent prostate cancer.

The hypothalamus normally releases gonadotropin-releasing hormone (GnRH) in a pulsatile fashion. Continuous administration of a GnRH analogue (the "relins") will suppress release of luteinizing hormone (LH) and follicle-stimulating hormone (FSH) and, as a result, decrease estrogen and testosterone levels, but there may be an initial surge in hormone levels before the decline. Antagonists of GnRH receptors will have the same effect but will cause an immediate decrease in hormone levels. The GnRH analogues and antagonists are used in the treatment of androgen-dependent prostate cancer.

PATHWAY-TARGETED THERAPIES

The most recent approach to treatment of cancers includes targeting pathways with monoclonal antibodies (-mab) that recognize cell surface antigens and small molecules (-ib) that recognize intracellular targets, many of them kinases. This is a rapidly changing field, so any drug list here will be out of date when you see it.

GROWTH FACTORS AND RECEPTORS

Epidermal growth factor receptor belongs to the family of tyrosine kinase receptors that are essential for the growth and differentiation of epithelial cells. There are inhibitors of extracellular ligand binding (cetuximab, panitumumab, and necitumumab) and kinase inhibitors (erlotinib, gefitinib, afatinib, and osimertinib). There are also both antibody (TRASTUZUMAB and pertuzumab) and small molecule (lapatinib, neratinib, and tucatinib) inhibitors of HER2 (human epidermal growth factor 2). So far, there is one antibody to platelet-derived growth factor receptor.

INTRACELLULAR KINASES

Imatinib was the first kinase inhibitor to be developed. In some patients with chronic myelogenous leukemia, the chromosomal translocation (Philadelphia chromosome) results in the formation of a tyrosine kinase (BCR-ABL kinase) that the cell cannot regulate (constitutively active). Imatinib binds to the ATP site on the newly formed kinase and can stop the growth of cells that contain this abnormal kinase. Normal cells are not affected. It is also useful against gastrointestinal stromal tumors. The discovery of the imatinib opened the door to the testing and development of other kinase inhibitors for a variety of cancers. Notice the "nib" or "ib" ending of these names.

Inhibitors of RAF kinase	Inhibitors of BCR-ABL kinase
dabrafenib	bosutinib
encorafenib—BRAF kinase inhibitor	dasatinib
vemurafenib—BRAF kinase inhibitor	imatinib
Inhibitors of MEK—act downstream of RAF	nilotinib
binimetinib	ponatinib
cobimetinib	Inhibitors of the anaplastic lymphoma kinase (ALK)
trametinib	alectinib
Inhibitor of JAK1/2	ceritinib
ruxolitinib	crizotinib
Inhibitors of CDK 4/6 (-ciclib)	Inhibitors of the PI3K/Akt/mTOR pathway
abemaciclib	idelalisib
palbociclib	Rapamycins—everolimus/sirolimus/temsirolimus
ribociclib	
Inhibitors of BTK (Bruton tyrosine kinase)	Multikinase Inhibitors
acalabrutinib	cabozantinib
ibrutinib	midostaurin
	vandetanib

ANGIOGENESIS

Cancer cells can induce the formation of new blood vessels. Inhibition of a number of secreted angiogenic factors has become useful therapeutically. Inhibition of

VEGF (vascular epidermal growth factor) has become an important class of anti-tumor agents. Bevacizumab and ramucirumab interact with the receptor, while aflibercept acts as a trap for VEGF. There are also several inhibitors of the kinase function related to VEGF, including pazopanib, sorafenib, sunitinib, and axitinib.

OTHER TARGETS

Monoclonal antibodies that block CTLA-4, PD-1 or PD-L1 are currently used to neutralize receptors during T-cell priming. These antibodies enable T cells to recognize and eradicate cancer cells with acceptable adverse effects.

atezolizumab—PD-L1 (trials)	ipilimumab—CTLA-4
avelumab—PD-L1	nivolumab—PD-1
durvalumab—PD-L1	pembrolizumab—PD-1

Rituximab is an antibody to CD20, a protein expressed on ~90% of B-cell cancers.

MISCELLANEOUS AGENTS

Bortezomib is a proteasome inhibitor. The proteasome is a large complex of proteins that is responsible for the regulation of protein expression and the degradation of damaged or used proteins in the cell. Importantly, it regulates the expression of cell cycle proteins. Happily, malignant cells are more sensitive to inhibition of proteasome function than normal cells.

Agents such as retinoids stimulate the growth of normal myeloid and erythroid progenitors and cause differentiation of myeloid leukemia cells. Clinical trials have shown that transretinoic acid (tretinoin) induces remission in acute promyelocytic leukemia. BCL-2 is overexpressed in many cells in chronic lymphocytic leukemia, which results in increased tumor cell survival and resistance to chemotherapy. An oral selective BCL-2 inhibitor, venetoclax, is now available for treatment of CLL in patients with a 17p deletion.

A couple a histone deacetylase (HDAC) inhibitors (romidepsin and vorinostat) have been approved for the treatment of cutaneous T-cell lymphoma. HDAC inhibitors cause acetylated nuclear histones to accumulate in both tumor and normal tissues. In addition, acetylated transcription factors are also found.

PART VI Drugs That Affect the Endocrine System

CHAPTER 38:   Adrenocortical Hormones   193

CHAPTER 39:   Sex Steroids   197

CHAPTER 40:   Thyroid and Parathyroid Drugs   204

CHAPTER 41:   Insulin, Glucagon, and Oral Hypoglycemic Drugs   207

Adrenocortical Hormones

Organization of Class
Glucocorticoids
Mineralocorticoids
Inhibitors of Adrenocorticoid Synthesis

ORGANIZATION OF CLASS

Now would be a good time to do a quick review of the anatomy of the adrenal gland and the normal release of cortisol and aldosterone. Remember that the adrenal medulla produces epinephrine and norepinephrine. Within the adrenal cortex, there are three layers. The zona glomerulosa (outer layer) produces the compounds that control electrolyte balance, such as aldosterone. The zona fasciculata (middle layer) produces the compounds that regulate metabolism, such as hydrocortisone. The zona reticularis (inner layer) produces the sex hormones (see Chapter 39). The pituitary hormone adrenocorticotropic hormone (ACTH) controls the secretion of, primarily, the inner two layers. The production of mineralocorticoids is mainly controlled by the renin-angiotensin system.

Deficiency of the adrenocortical hormones results in the signs and symptoms of Addison disease. Excess production causes Cushing syndrome. Both natural and synthetic corticosteroids are used to diagnose and treat disorders of adrenal function and treat a variety of inflammatory and immunologic disorders.

The term *steroid* relates to the main structural frame of this series of compounds (Figure 38–1).

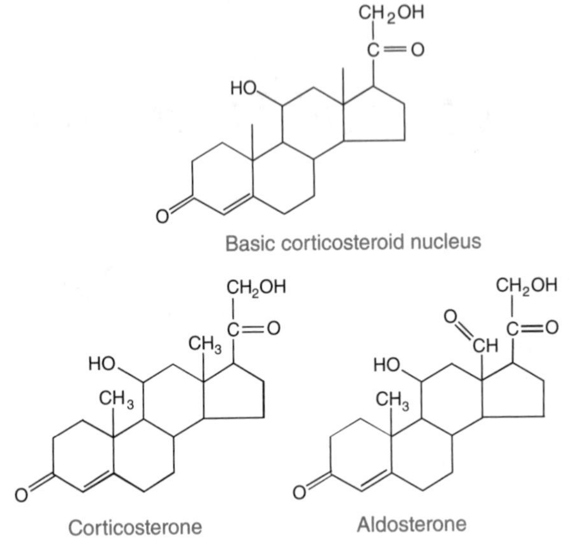

FIGURE 38-1 The main steroid structure is shown, along with two examples of adrenocortical hormones.

The steroid compounds produced by the adrenal cortex are called *adrenocorticosteroids*, and they can be divided into two main groups depending on their relative metabolic (glucocorticoid) versus electrolyte-regulating (mineralocorticoid) activity. Of course, each compound has effects on both metabolism and electrolyte balance, but one effect is usually more potent than the other. Almost every cell in the body will respond to these compounds.

Glucocorticoid	Equal Potency	Mineralocorticoid
DEXAMETHASONE	cortisol	fludrocortisone
PREDNISONE	hydrocortisone	
fluticasone		
betamethasone		
methylprednisolone		
prednisolone		
triamcinolone		

Compare this list of drugs with the list in your textbook or class handouts and make any necessary changes. I have found lists of more than 20 glucocorticoids, so the table above is quite abbreviated. You may also find a list dividing the drugs into short, intermediate, and long acting. This is useful information to add if you have time.

Hydrocortisone (cortisol) is the main glucocorticoid, and aldosterone is the main mineralocorticoid produced by the adrenal glands. Notice that hydrocortisone and its close relative, cortisol, are the *only* two drugs that have equal metabolic (glucocorticoid) and electrolyte balance (mineralocorticoid) actions. Remember this. Next, notice that there are many more drugs listed on the left (glucocorticoid) than on the right (mineralocorticoid). Therefore, if you have to guess about the activity of a drug, guess glucocorticoid. Better yet, just learn the mineralocorticoid drug on the right (it starts with "f," but it's not the only one that does).

> The pharmacologic actions of steroids are an extension of their physiological effects.

This should seem self-evident, but sometimes it is forgotten.

> All of the steroids (including the sex steroids) bind to intracellular receptors in target tissues.

After entering the cell and binding to the receptor, the receptor-hormone complex is transported into the nucleus where it acts as a transcription factor for specific genes. The actions of the glucocorticoids and mineralocorticoids will be reviewed separately.

GLUCOCORTICOIDS

Glucocorticoid receptors are found in virtually every cell in the body.

> Glucocorticoids promote catabolism of proteins and gluconeogenesis.

The glucocorticoids stimulate formation of glucose and cause breakdown of proteins into amino acids. The net effect is to increase liver glycogen levels, fasting blood glucose levels, and urinary nitrogen output.

> Glucocorticoids inhibit inflammatory and immunologic responses. This is the basis of their therapeutic use and the reason why patients on glucocorticoids have increased susceptibility to infections.

Glucocorticoids are used for replacement therapy in patients with malfunctioning adrenal glands. But the most important use of glucocorticoids is to reduce inflammation or block immunological and allergic responses. All steps in the inflammatory process are blocked.

Glucocorticoids have a number of other actions. You should read about them, but do not try to memorize them early on.

> The complications of glucocorticoid therapy appear in all organ systems.

This should be intuitive. Because the glucocorticoids affect nearly every cell in the body, the adverse effects can arise from nearly every cell in the body.

Short-term use (e.g., in status asthmaticus) is generally safe. It is long-term use that poses particular problems.

> A potentially serious complication of long-term use is osteoporosis.

Glucocorticoids affect bone metabolism in a number of ways. The final result is a decrease in calcification. With long-term therapy, redistribution of fat also occurs, resulting in truncal obesity, moon facies, and buffalo hump. The effects on protein metabolism cause delayed wound healing.

> When possible, glucocorticoids should be dosed on alternate days. Therapy should not be decreased or stopped abruptly. When the dose needs to be decreased, it should be tapered slowly.

When administered for more than 2 weeks, glucocorticoids may suppress adrenal function and it takes time for it to recover.

MINERALOCORTICOIDS

> Mineralocorticoids are involved in salt and water balance.

Mineralocorticoids increase the rate of sodium, bicarbonate, and water reabsorption and potassium excretion. These actions help maintain normal concentrations of sodium and potassium in the serum.

INHIBITORS OF ADRENOCORTICOID SYNTHESIS

This group of drugs is used clinically to treat the glucocorticoid overproduction that appears in some diseases (Cushing disease, adrenal carcinoma, and others).

Osilodrostat is an orally active cortisol synthesis inhibitor for the treatment of adults with Cushing disease. Metyrapone and aminoglutethimide are used off-label to inhibit adrenocorticoid synthesis. Name recognition is the most important thing here. If you have the time and energy, add the mechanisms of action. All three drugs inhibit the conversion of cholesterol to pregnenolone by an enzyme called 11-β-hydroxylase (the rate-limiting step in steroid synthesis).

Ketoconazole, an antifungal agent, and spironolactone, an antagonist of aldosterone, also inhibit adrenal hormone synthesis.

Sex Steroids

CHAPTER

39

- Organization of Class
- Estrogens
- Antiestrogens
- Progestins
- Antiprogestins
- Oral Contraceptives
- Androgens
- Antiandrogens
- GnRH Agonists and Antagonists
- PDE5 Inhibitors

ORGANIZATION OF CLASS

Sex hormones are produced by the gonads and inner layer of the cortex of the adrenal medulla. The synthesis and release of the hormones are controlled by the anterior pituitary (luteinizing hormone [LH] and follicle-stimulating hormone [FSH]) and the hypothalamus (gonadotropin-releasing hormone [GnRH]). Therefore, we include in this chapter the actual sex steroids, but also GnRH agonists and antagonists.

Estrogens	Antiestrogens
DIETHYLSTILBESTROL	CLOMIPHENE
ESTRADIOL	TAMOXIFEN (SERM)
estriol	RALOXIFENE (SERM)
estrone	toremifene (SERM)
ethinyl estradiol	
mestranol	
quinestrol	

(Continued)

Progestins	Antiprogestins
PROGESTERONE	MIFEPRISTONE
hydroxyprogesterone	
medroxyprogesterone	
megestrol	
norethindrone	
norgestrel	
levonorgestrel	

Androgens	Antiandrogens
TESTOSTERONE	dutasteride (5α-*reductase inhibitor*)
(several preparations)	FINASTERIDE (5α-*reductase inhibitor*)
fluoxymesterone	bicalutamide (*receptor antagonist*)
	flutamide (*receptor antagonist*)
methyltestosterone	nilutamide (*receptor antagonist*)
testolactone	cyproterone acetate

First, compare these drug names to those in your textbook or class handouts. The androgens listed here are only the androgenic steroids. I have not included the agents used primarily as anabolic agents. Look at each name and decide whether you recognize it for what it is. (That is, do you know that norgestrel is a progestin?) Put those you are not sure of in your list for name recognition. The rest of this is easy, especially if you remember your physiology.

As with the glucocorticoids, the sex steroids bind to specific intracellular receptors that are nuclear transcription factors.

ESTROGENS

> The major estrogens produced by the body are estradiol, estrone, and estriol.

The ovary is the primary source of estradiol. Estrone and estriol are metabolites of estradiol, courtesy of the liver.

> The most common use of estrogens is in oral contraceptives.

Estrogen therapy combined with progestins is used to block ovulation and prevent pregnancy. In postmenopausal women, estrogens can be used to reduce the symptoms of menopause and osteoporosis. Hormone replacement therapies can slow bone loss but cannot reverse existing deficits. However, there is now evidence that the risks of estrogen-replacement therapy may outweigh the benefits.

> The most common side effects of estrogens are nausea and vomiting.

Estrogens can also cause breast tenderness, endometrial hyperplasia, hyperpigmentation, edema (sodium and water retention), and weight gain.

> DIETHYLSTILBESTROL (a nonsteroid molecule) has been associated with cervical and vaginal carcinoma in daughters of women who took the drug during pregnancy.

ANTIESTROGENS

There are two important groups of drugs that antagonize the action of estrogen—the selective estrogen receptor modulators (SERMs) and clomiphene.

> The selective estrogen receptor modulators (SERMs) are not pure antagonists but mixed agonists/antagonists.

Tamoxifen and toremifene are used in the prevention and treatment of breast cancer that has estrogen receptors. These drugs are antagonists in breast tissue and partial agonists in bone and endometrial tissue. Raloxifene has agonist activity in bone, but antagonist activity in breast and endometrial tissue. Raloxifene and bazedoxifene are approved for treatment of postmenopausal osteoporosis (see Chapter 47).

> CLOMIPHENE stimulates ovarian function and is used in the treatment of infertility.

Clomiphene acts as an estrogen receptor antagonist in the hypothalamus, thus interfering with the inhibitory feedback of estrogens. This results in an increase in release of gonadotropin-releasing hormone and gonadotropins and in stimulation of ovarian function.

PROGESTINS

> PROGESTERONE is the main natural progestin.

Progesterone is produced in the corpus luteum and placenta. Its job is to maintain the uterine endometrium in the secretory phase.

> The major use of progestins is in oral contraceptives.

Other clinical uses of progestins include dysfunctional uterine bleeding, suppression of postpartum lactation, treatment of dysmenorrhea, and management of endometriosis.

> The most common side effects of progestin use are weight gain, edema, and depression.

Increased clotting may also occur, leading to thrombophlebitis or pulmonary embolism.

ANTIPROGESTINS

> MIFEPRISTONE is an antiprogestin that works to terminate pregnancy by breaking down the uterine lining.

The current regimen for medical abortion is a multistep process. Mifepristone is administered first, followed 2 days later by misoprostol (see Chapter 44). As an antiprogestin, mifepristone can also be used to treat cases of infertility, endometriosis, and some tumors. It also has potential as a contraceptive.

ORAL CONTRACEPTIVES

> The most common pharmacological means of preventing pregnancy is the use of estrogens and progestins to interfere with ovulation.

The mechanism of action of the oral contraceptives is not completely understood. The estrogen provides negative feedback to the pituitary, inhibiting further release of LH and FSH. This prevents ovulation. The progestin also inhibits LH and is added to stimulate withdrawal bleeding.

> Progestin alone in pill form (mini-pill) or implants also provides contraception.

The use of progestin alone is associated with irregular uterine bleeding.

> The side effects of the oral contraceptives are related to the estrogens and progestins that are part of the pills.

I hope you said "Wait, that's obvious!" The major side effects of the combination pills are breast fullness, nausea and vomiting (estrogen), depression, and edema (progestin). There is an increased incidence of abnormal clotting in women who smoke and are over the age of 35.

ANDROGENS

The androgens have masculinizing and anabolic effects in both men and women. The anabolic effects include increased muscle mass, increased bone density, and increased red blood cell mass. The virilizing effects include spermatogenesis, sexual dysfunction, or restoration and development of male characteristics. It is possible to separate (somewhat) the virilizing and anabolic activities by altering the structure of the steroid.

> TESTOSTERONE is the major androgen produced in the body.

Testosterone is produced by the Leydig cells of the testes and by the ovaries and adrenal glands. The secretion of testosterone is controlled by hormonal signals from the hypothalamus and anterior pituitary.

> The primary therapeutic use of androgens is for replacement therapy in patients with testicular deficiency.

Although the most common use of the androgens is for replacement therapy, androgens can be used to stimulate linear bone growth and in the treatment of anemia.

> The side effects of the androgens are related to their physiological actions.

This is simple enough. Androgens cause virilization of women, including acne, growth of facial hair, deepening of the voice, and excessive muscle development. In men, androgens can cause impotence, decreased spermatogenesis, gynecomastia, liver abnormalities, and psychotic episodes. In children, androgens cause closure of epiphyseal plates and abnormal sexual maturation. These should all make sense and do not need to be memorized.

ANTIANDROGENS

Competitive antagonists of testosterone include cyproterone acetate and flutamide. These drugs have been used to treat excessive hair growth in women and prostate cancer in men.

> FINASTERIDE is a 5α-reductase inhibitor that is used to treat cases of benign prostatic hypertrophy (and to stimulate hair growth).

5α-Reductase converts testosterone to dihydrotestosterone. Dihydrotestosterone is the major intracellular androgen in most target tissues. Finasteride and dutasteride (note the similar names) are effective in slowing the growth of prostate tissue without interfering with libido (mediated by testosterone).

GnRH AGONISTS AND ANTAGONISTS

Under physiologic conditions, the hypothalamus releases GnRH (also called LH-RH) in a pulsatile manner. The frequency of the pulses controls the release of LH and FSH by the anterior pituitary.

> The hypothalamic-pituitary-gonadal axis can be suppressed by administration of either a gonadotropin-releasing hormone (GnRH) agonist or an antagonist.

At first this doesn't make sense but remember that GnRH release is pulsatile. Continuous administration of a GnRH agonist will suppress release of LH and FSH by desensitizing the pituitary to the activity of GnRH. The GnRH agonists, which (almost) all end in "relin," can be used in prostate cancer, endometriosis, and precocious puberty because of their suppression of estrogen and testosterone levels. Beware of an initial flare (release of LH and FSH) in the first 7 to 10 days.

GnRH Agonists and Analogues	GnRH Antagonists
triptorelin	abarelix
nafarelin	cetrorelix
goserelin	degarelix
histrelin	ganirelix
leuprolide	

The GnRH antagonists (the "relix"s) competitively block GnRH receptors in the pituitary without causing receptor desensitization. This results in suppression of LH and FSH secretion from the anterior pituitary. Cetrorelix and ganirelix are used to inhibit premature LH surges in women undergoing fertility treatments. Abarelix is used in advanced prostate cancer.

PDE5 INHIBITORS

No, these drugs are not sex steroids, but there was no good place in the book to put them. Short of making a chapter just for one class, this seemed like as good a place as any. These drugs are orally active agents used in the treatment of erectile dysfunction.

Avanafil, sildenafil, tadalafil, and vardenafil inhibit a phosphodiesterase found in vascular smooth muscle.

Nitric oxide is released from nerve endings and endothelial cells. It binds to receptors on the smooth muscle of the corpus cavernosum and triggers the formation of cyclic guanosine monophosphate (cGMP). cGMP causes relaxation of smooth muscle, allowing engorgement. This process is reversed by a phosphodiesterase (number 5) that converts the cGMP to GMP. These drugs inhibit this phosphodiesterase.

All of these drugs potentiate the hypotensive action of nitrates. Their use together with nitrates could result in a fatal drop in blood pressure. Interestingly, sildenafil and tadalafil are also approved for the treatment of pulmonary arterial hypertension (see Chapter 43).

40 Thyroid and Parathyroid Drugs

Organization of Class
Thyroid Replacement Therapy
Drugs That Are Thyroid Downers
Parathyroid Drugs

ORGANIZATION OF CLASS

These drugs are really quite simple if you can recognize the names and if you remember how the thyroid gland is controlled and how it synthesizes thyroid hormone (Figure 40–1).

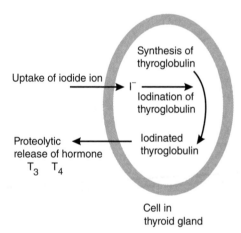

FIGURE 40–1 In each thyroid cell there is active uptake of iodide. This iodide is then incorporated onto tyrosine residues in the protein thyroglobulin. The iodinated thyroglobulin then undergoes proteolysis to release thyroid hormone in the form of triiodothyronine (T_3) and thyroxine (T_4).

The thyroid gland helps regulate metabolism in tissues. Hypothyroidism (low levels of hormone) results in slow heart rate (bradycardia), cold intolerance, and physical slowing. In children, hypothyroidism can result in mental retardation and short stature. Hyperthyroidism (too much hormone) results in fast heart rate, nervousness, tremor, and excess heat production.

> The thyroid gland stores thyroid hormone as thyroglobulin.

THYROID REPLACEMENT THERAPY

The most common cause of hypothyroidism is iodine deficiency, which is treated with iodine. The most common cause of hypothyroidism in the United States is probably Hashimoto thyroiditis, an immunologic disorder.

> There are two major thyroid hormones, called T_3 (triiodothyronine) and T_4 (thyroxine).

Thyroxine (T_4) is the major secretory product of the thyroid gland. Triiodo-thyronine (T_3) is secreted by the thyroid but is also synthesized by extrathyroid metabolism of T_4. Both T_4 and T_3 are bound to thyroxine-binding globulin and several other proteins in the plasma. T_4 is often referred to as thyroxine and T_3 as triiodothyronine.

> LEVOTHYROXINE (a sodium salt of T_4) is the *drug of choice* for the treatment of hypothyroidism.

Liothyronine (a sodium salt of T_3) and liotrix (a mixture of T_3 and T_4) have also been used to treat hypothyroidism.

DRUGS THAT ARE THYROID DOWNERS

Treatment of hyperthyroidism is achieved by removing part, or all, of the thyroid gland, inhibiting synthesis of thyroid hormone, or by blocking release of hormone from the gland.

> Surgery or radioactive iodine can be used to destroy the thyroid gland.

Remember that iodine is taken up selectively by the thyroid gland. Therefore, administration of radioactive iodine will result in the accumulation of radioactivity in the thyroid gland. This is very selective radiation therapy.

> PROPYLTHIOURACIL and METHIMAZOLE inhibit thyroid synthesis.

Propylthiouracil and methimazole inhibit iodination of tyrosine groups and coupling of these groups to form thyroid hormone. They have no effect on the stored thyroglobulin or on the release of thyroid hormone. Therefore, there will be a delay between the onset of therapy and the clinical effect as the previously stored thyroglobulin is released. Propylthiouracil also inhibits the peripheral conversion of T_4 to T_3. Propylthiouracil causes severe hepatic toxicity.

Note that methimazole ends in—azole, but it is NOT an antifungal agent.

β-Blockers without intrinsic sympathomimetic activity (not partial agonists) can improve symptoms of thyrotoxicosis but do not lower hormone levels.

PARATHYROID DRUGS

The most important endocrine regulator of calcium homeostasis is parathyroid hormone (PTH), which is secreted by the parathyroid gland.

> High serum calcium suppresses parathyroid hormone (PTH) secretion and low serum calcium stimulates PTH release.

PTH acts directly on the kidney to increase calcium reabsorption and on the bone to increase bone mass, while acting indirectly on the gastrointestinal (GI) tract to improve calcium absorption.

> Teriparatide (peptides 1-34) and natpara (full length peptide) are recombinant parathyroid hormones used for replacement therapy.

Teriparatide is also used for treatment of osteoporosis.

Hyperparathyroidism is commonly treated with a synthetic vitamin D analogue, such as paricalcitol and doxercalciferol, or surgery.

> Cinacalcet increases the sensitivity of calcium-sensing receptors in the parathyroid gland resulting in a decrease in PTH and serum calcium levels.

Cinacalcet can be used in the management of secondary hyperparathyroidism in patients with chronic renal failure on dialysis and in the treatment of hypercalcemia due to a parathyroid tumor.

Insulin, Glucagon, and Oral Hypoglycemic Drugs

Organization of Class

Insulins

Oral Hypoglycemic Agents

    Stimulation of Insulin Release

    Decrease Production of Glucose

    Increase Sensitivity of Tissues to What Insulin Is Available

    Reduce Absorption of Glucose

    Increase Elimination of Glucose

ORGANIZATION OF CLASS

A high level of glucose stimulates an increase in insulin release from β cells of the pancreas. Insulin then drives carbohydrate into cells. Patients who have high glucose levels in their blood are said to have diabetes mellitus.

Of course, you remember that diabetes mellitus is divided into two groups: type 1 (insulin dependent) and type 2 (insulin resistant). These distinctions are important for pharmacology because they make it easier to remember the mechanism of action of the drugs used to treat diabetes mellitus.

As an aside, there is another form of diabetes that students sometimes confuse with diabetes mellitus and that is diabetes insipidus. Diabetes insipidus is a disorder of water and sodium balance. Generally, if someone says *diabetes,* they mean the sugar-related (mellitus) disease and not diabetes insipidus.

But let's return to the topic at hand.

> Type 1 diabetes is related to loss of insulin-secreting cells in the pancreas. Type 2 diabetes is related to target cell resistance to the action of insulin.

This, of course, is somewhat simplified. An endocrinologist would cringe. Patients with type 1 diabetes are dependent on an exogenous (outside the body) source of insulin. This disorder generally appears in childhood; hence, the former term for it is *juvenile diabetes.* Type 2 diabetes has been called *adult-onset.* It appears to have a genetic basis, and patients are often obese. Patients with type 2 diabetes are treated with oral agents that lower blood glucose (hypoglycemics) and with insulin.

So, that said, we should organize our drugs into insulins and the oral hypoglycemic agents.

INSULINS

Insulin is a small protein that is synthesized and secreted by the β cells of the pancreas. Insulin for replacement therapy can be isolated from animal sources. Human insulin is made using recombinant DNA technology.

> INSULIN must be administered by injection and doses are expressed in international units of activity.

All peptides are degraded by enzymes in the gastrointestinal (GI) tract, so it is not possible to administer insulin by the oral route. Given intravenously, it has a half-life of less than 10 minutes (short). Therefore, it is administered subcutaneously.

> The most common adverse effect of insulin is hypoglycemia.

I hope that this is intuitively obvious.

> Insulin preparations vary in their time to onset and duration of action.

The onset and duration of action of the insulin preparations are controlled by the size and composition of the crystals in the particular insulin preparation.

Types of Insulin Preparations
Rapid onset and short duration
aspart
lispro
insulin glulisine
crystalline zinc insulin (regular)
prompt insulin (SEMILENTE)
Intermediate onset and duration
isophane insulin (NPH)
insulin zinc (LENTE, mixture of semilente and ultralente)
Prolonged duration
protamine zinc insulin
extended insulin zinc (ULTRALENTE)
insulin degludec
insulin detemir
insulin glargine

Basically, insulin is crystallized as a zinc salt. That's where the zinc comes from. When zinc is added to the solution, the molecules of insulin associate. These larger molecules diffuse more slowly. The rapidly acting analogues, lispro and aspart, are formulated to dissociate rapidly. The protamine is a positively charged peptide mixture that delays the absorption of the insulin (less soluble complex). In other words, reducing the solubility decreases the absorption and increases the duration of action. Insulin detemir reversibly binds to albumin, which increases its duration of action. Just as an aside, NPH stands for neutral protamine Hagedorn.

Combinations of short- and long-acting insulins reduce the number of daily injections.

ORAL HYPOGLYCEMIC AGENTS

The oral hypoglycemic agents are so named because they lower blood glucose (hypoglycemic) and can be administered orally (as opposed to insulin). That makes the route of administration easy to remember. These drugs are organized in different ways by different textbooks. Look and see how your book or class organizes them.

STIMULATION OF INSULIN RELEASE

Sulfonylureas (2nd)	GLP-1 Agonists	DPP-4 inhibitors
glimepiride	albiglutide	alogliptin
glipizide	dulaglutide	linagliptin
glyburide	liraglutide	saxagliptin
	exenatide (analogue)	sitagliptin
Meglitinides (Glinides)	lixisenatide	
nateglinide	semaglutide	
repaglinide		

> The sulfonylureas act by stimulating the release of insulin from the β cells in the pancreas by an interaction with the ATP-sensitive potassium channels.

The sulfonylureas stimulate insulin release, reduce serum glucagon levels, and increase binding of insulin to target tissues. Historically, the sulfonylureas were divided into two groups: first generation and second generation. The first-generation drugs are rarely used anymore having been replaced by the second-generation drugs. The drugs vary in their duration of action and side effects. For now, name recognition is the most important thing for you to focus on.

Nateglinide and repaglinide bind to the ATP-sensitive potassium channels on the β cells to increase insulin release, but are not structurally sulfonylureas, hence the categorization as nonsulfonylureas secretagogues.

> The most common adverse effect of the sulfonylureas and meglitinides is hypoglycemia.

I hope you can remember that without too much problem.

> Exenatide and the "-glutides" are peptide GLP agonists that stimulate insulin release, inhibit glucagon release, delay gastric emptying, and reduce food intake.

Exenatide and the "-glutides" are peptides similar to the incretin hormone glucagon-like peptide-1 (GLP-1), which, in the presence of glucose, acts to stimulate insulin secretion.

> The dipeptidyl-peptidase-4 (DPP-4) inhibitors increase insulin secretion, reduce glucagon levels, and improve both fasting and postprandial hyperglycemia. These drugs are orally bioavailable.

Sitagliptin and relatives are called dipeptidyl-peptidase-4 (DPP-4) inhibitors. DPP-4 is responsible for inactivation and degradation of two GI hormones that lower serum glucose production, GLP-1 and glucose-dependent insulinotropic polypeptide (GIP). These GI hormones potentiate insulin synthesis and release by β cells in the pancreas and decrease glucagon production by α cells. When you inhibit the degradation of these hormones, they can continue to lower serum glucose.

DECREASE PRODUCTION OF GLUCOSE

> Metformin is an orally active hypoglycemic that is currently first line therapy for type 2 diabetes. A rare, but often listed and potentially fatal, side effect is lactic acidosis, particularly in patients with renal impairment.

Metformin is considered a "biguanide." It decreases glucose output from the liver and increases peripheral glucose utilization. It is effective as monotherapy and is useful in combination with other glucose-lowering drugs.

INCREASE SENSITIVITY OF TISSUES TO WHAT INSULIN IS AVAILABLE

> The "-glitazones," such as rosiglitazone and pioglitazone, are orally active and increase sensitivity to insulin.

The "-glitazones" are thiazolidinediones (TZDs). These drugs enhance the action of insulin at target tissues by acting as agonists for the nuclear hormone receptor called *peroxisome proliferator activated receptor-gamma* (PPAR-γ). PPAR-γ regulates the production of proteins involved in glucose and lipid metabolism. There is ongoing concern about possible increased risk of heart failure in patients on these drugs.

REDUCE ABSORPTION OF GLUCOSE

The α-glucosidase inhibitors (acarbose, miglitol, and voglibose) are nicknamed the "starch blockers." They increase the time required for absorption of carbohydrates, thus reducing the peak glucose levels after eating. They will not reduce hyperglycemia at other times.

INCREASE ELIMINATION OF GLUCOSE

Sodium-glucose co-transporter 2 (SGLT2) is a membrane protein in the kidney that transports filtered glucose from the renal tubule into epithelial cells. Inhibition of this transporter reduces glucose reabsorption and increases glucose excretion. The result is lowering of blood glucose levels and a modest reduction in hemoglobin A_{1c} (HbA_{1c}).

> The "-gliflozins," canagliflozin, dapagliflozin, empagliflozin, reduce A_{1c}, cause weight loss, and decrease blood pressure.

Pramlintide is a synthetic analogue of amylin, a small peptide hormone that is released into the bloodstream by the β cells of the pancreas along with insulin. Amylin reduces the production of glucose by the liver by inhibiting the action of glucagon.

PART VII Miscellaneous Drugs

CHAPTER 42:   Histamine and Antihistamines   215

CHAPTER 43:   Respiratory Drugs   217

CHAPTER 44:   Drugs That Affect the GI Tract   222

CHAPTER 45:   Nonnarcotic Analgesics and Anti-inflammatory Drugs   227

CHAPTER 46:   Immunosuppressives   234

CHAPTER 47:   Drugs Used in Osteoporosis   236

CHAPTER 48:   Toxicology and Poisoning   239

Histamine and Antihistamines

Organization of Class
H$_1$ Receptor Antagonists

ORGANIZATION OF CLASS

Histamine is an endogenous substance that is widely distributed throughout the body. The two principal sites of storage for histamine are the mast cells in tissue and the basophils in blood.

> The action of histamine is mediated through at least two receptors, H$_1$ and H$_2$.

H$_3$ receptors have been reported in the brain, but for our purposes there are two classes of histamine receptors.

> Intestinal and bronchial smooth muscles contain mostly H$_1$ receptors. Gastric secretion is mediated by H$_2$ receptors.

As you can see, the action of histamine depends on the receptors with which it interacts. Histamine itself or agonists of the histamine receptors have only minor uses in clinical medicine. Because we consider drugs that act on the gastrointestinal (GI) tract in Chapter 44, we will not consider the H$_2$ receptor antagonists any further here.

H$_1$ RECEPTOR ANTAGONISTS

H$_1$ Receptor Antagonists	
DIPHENHYDRAMINE	chlorpheniramine
acrivastine	dimenhydrinate
azelastine	hydroxyzine
brompheniramine	meclizine
clemastine	promethazine

(Continued)

H₁ Receptor Antagonists (*Continued*)	
cyclizine	
cyproheptadine	
olopatadine	
Nonsedating Antihistamines	
astemizole	fexofenadine
cetirizine	levocetirizine
desloratadine	loratadine

As always, compare this list with the one in your textbook or class handouts and make any adjustments. Some books will divide these drugs into first- and second-generation H_1 antihistamines, or into sedating versus nonsedating groups. Second-generation antihistamines do not cross into the brain as easily as the first-generation drugs and are, therefore, less likely to have central nervous system (CNS) side effects. Because many of the first-generation drugs are available over the counter, they are more recognizable by their trade names. They are inexpensive, but have significant side effects, including sedation and anticholinergic effects.

> These drugs are competitive antagonists of the H_1 receptor.

> The H_1 antagonists (antihistamines) are used to treat cases of allergic rhinitis and motion sickness, and sometimes to induce sleep.

First, note that this class of drugs is commonly referred as antihistamines. This is in spite of the fact that there is a whole group of H_2 antagonists that could also be called antihistamines but aren't.

The most common use of antihistamines is in the treatment of runny nose caused by seasonal allergies. The first-generation drugs cross the blood-brain barrier. In the CNS, they interact with histamine receptors and cause sedation. This effect is sometimes used therapeutically. A number of these drugs are used to treat motion sickness (diphenhydramine, dimenhydrinate, cyclizine, and meclizine). This action may be the result of a central antihistamine effect or a central anticholinergic action. The agents in this class vary in terms of their anticholinergic potency, the degree of sedation they induce, and their duration of action.

> The nonsedating antihistamines (second generation) do not cross the blood-brain barrier, so are less sedating.

Be absolutely sure you know the names of these second-generation nonsedating antihistamines. These are first-line therapy for mild to moderate allergic rhinitis.

Respiratory Drugs

43

Organization of Class
Bronchodilators
  β-Agonists
  Cholinergic Antagonists
  Methylxanthines
Anti-inflammatory Drugs
  Inhaled Corticosteroids
  PDE-4 Inhibitor
Other Approaches
  Leukotriene Modifiers
  Anti-IgE Therapy
  Other Biologics and Cromolyn
Pulmonary Hypertension
Cystic Fibrosis

ORGANIZATION OF CLASS

Bronchoconstriction, inflammation, and loss of lung elasticity are the most common processes that result in respiratory compromise. Bronchoconstriction can be treated with adrenergic agonists, cholinergic antagonists, and some other compounds. Inflammation is treatable with corticosteroids. Obstruction of the airways can also occur with infection and increased secretions. The infection is treated with antibiotics. Because the antibiotics and steroids have been covered elsewhere, this chapter focuses on the bronchodilators. Much of this will be a review from autonomic pharmacology.

> For asthma, emphasis is on inhaled steroids (anti-inflammatory). For chronic obstructive pulmonary disease (COPD), emphasis is on bronchodilation.

Most of these drugs are now administered by inhalation. This gets the drug to the site of action and limits the systemic effects.

BRONCHODILATORS

β-AGONISTS

> β_2-Agonists cause bronchodilation.

Inhaled short-acting β_2-agonists are the most effective drugs available for treatment of acute bronchospasm and for prevention of exercise-induced asthma. β_2-Selective agents are preferred to avoid the cardiac effect of β_1-activation.

There are a number of β-agonists that are used in the treatment of asthma and chronic obstructive pulmonary disease (COPD).

β-Agonists Used as Bronchodilators	
ALBUTEROL (SA)	arformoterol (LA)
levalbuterol (SA)	formoterol (LA)
	olodaterol (LA)
	salmeterol (LA)
SA, short-acting; LA, long acting	

In an emergency, such as the bronchoconstriction associated with anaphylaxis, epinephrine can be used. Use of a short-acting β-agonist more than two to three times a week means that the asthma is not well controlled and adjustments to baseline medication need to be made. Long-acting β-agonists can be used in combination with inhaled corticosteroids to control asthma symptoms.

CHOLINERGIC ANTAGONISTS

The cholinergic antagonists block the bronchoconstriction caused by activation of the parasympathetic nervous system.

> IPRATROPIUM (short-acting) and tiotropium (long-acting) are anticholinergic agents used for the treatment of COPD in adults.

The long-acting cholinergic antagonists, aclidinium, glycopyrrolate, revefenacin, tiotropium, and umeclidinium, have found use in the treatment of COPD. The anticholinergic drugs reduce air trapping and improve exercise tolerance in patients with COPD.

METHYLXANTHINES

Theophylline (or aminophylline) was once the treatment of choice for the management of asthma. Now, the combination of inhaled corticosteroids and β_2-agonists are first-line therapy. The methylxanthines increase cyclic adenosine monophosphate (cAMP) levels, but the exact mechanism by which they cause bronchodilation is not known. Theophylline is still listed as a treatment option for COPD. It is rare that students mistake these drugs for another class of compounds. The ending "-phylline" is a dead giveaway.

ANTI-INFLAMMATORY DRUGS

INHALED CORTICOSTEROIDS

> Inhaled corticosteroids used in the treatment of asthma include:
>
> | | |
> |---|---|
> | beclomethasone | fluticasone |
> | budesonide | mometasone |
> | ciclesonide | triamcinolone |

Inhaled corticosteroids reduce inflammation in the bronchial tree. Data suggest that use of a β_2 agonist together with an inhaled corticosteroid has synergistic activity.

PDE-4 INHIBITOR

Phosphodiesterase-4 inhibitors relax smooth muscle and inhibit inflammatory cells through an increase in cAMP. Roflumilast is approved for the treatment of severe COPD.

OTHER APPROACHES

LEUKOTRIENE MODIFIERS

Leukotriene modifiers can be used as add-on therapy for patients not well controlled with an inhaled corticosteroid. Montelukast and zafirlukast block binding of LTD_4 (the predominant cysteinyl leukotriene in the airways) to its receptor, thus decreasing mucus production, airway wall edema and bronchoconstriction. Zileuton inhibits leukotriene synthesis by inhibiting 5-lipoxygenase, which catalyzes the conversion of arachidonic acid to leukotrienes. These drugs are effective in preventing exercise-induced asthma.

ANTI-IGE THERAPY

> Omalizumab is a monoclonal antibody that blocks binding of IgE to its receptors on mast cells reducing circulating levels of IgE.

You should already know that omalizumab is a monoclonal antibody that must be administered by injection because the name ends in "mab." It binds to IgE's high-affinity Fc receptor, lowering the serum concentration of free IgE and preventing binding of IgE to a variety of cells, including mast cells. This will prevent activation (and degranulation) of these cells.

OTHER BIOLOGICS AND CROMOLYN

Interleukin-5 (IL-5) antibodies, benralizumab, mepolizumab, and reslizumab, will also reduce inflammation by binding to IL-5 and blocking its binding to the IL-5 receptor on the surface of eosinophils. Since IL-5 is the major cytokine involved in growth, differentiation, and activation of eosinophils, it makes sense that inhibiting the action of IL-5 will reduce production of eosinophils and reduce airway inflammation. These IL-5 antibodies have been shown to reduce asthma exacerbations, improve lung function and reduce the need for oral steroids.

IL-4 and IL-13 promote production of IgE and recruit inflammatory cells. Dupilumab can be given subcutaneously to treat atopic dermatitis and asthma by its interactions with IL-4 and IL-13

> CROMOLYN sodium is used prophylactically in the treatment of asthma.

Cromolyn is *not* useful in the treatment of an acute attack and is infrequently used these days. The mechanism of action of cromolyn is not clear. It does block the release of mediators from mast cells, but the relevance of this action has been questioned.

PULMONARY HYPERTENSION

Pulmonary arterial hypertension (PAH) is an uncommon disease characterized by increased pulmonary artery pressure and vascular resistance. The predominant symptom is shortness of breath—hence it's included in the chapter on respiratory drugs. Data indicate that inflammation has a prominent role in the pathogenesis of PAH. Also, endothelin-1 levels are increased in plasma and lung tissue of patients with PAH, suggesting a role of endothelin-1 in the pathogenesis.

> Endothelin-receptor antagonists (ambrisentan, bosentan, and macitentan) and prostacyclin analogues (epoprostenol, iloprost, and treprostinil) or agonists (selexipag) are available for use in pulmonary hypertension.

Bosentan is a specific and competitive antagonist of both types A and B endothelin-1 receptors, while ambrisentan is specific for type A receptors. Both can improve exercise ability and slow the progression of the disease. Bosentan lowers systemic vascular resistance, pulmonary vascular resistance, and mean pulmonary arterial pressure. Both of these drugs can be given orally. The PDE5 inhibitors (sildenafil and tadalafil), which increase levels of cGMP, can also be used for PAH. A soluble guanylate cyclase stimulator (riociguat) is also approved for use in pulmonary hypertension.

The prostacyclin analogues are reserved for more advanced disease, in part because they must be given by injection.

CYSTIC FIBROSIS

Cystic fibrosis is not just a respiratory disease, but because of the changes in mucus consistency the main symptoms are respiratory. The genetic defect alters the function of a regulated chloride channel called the cystic fibrosis transmembrane conductance regulator (CFTR). At least five classes of cystic fibrosis mutations have been identified to organize the more than 1900 identified mutations. The F508del mutation, which occurs in about 50% of patients in the United States, causes the protein to misfold. Lumacaftor, tezacaftor, and elexacaftor improve the conformational stability of the protein increasing the number of CFTR proteins that make it to the cell surface. They are used in combination with ivacaftor which increases chloride transport through the channel.

44 Drugs That Affect the GI Tract

Organization of Class
Drugs That Act in the Upper GI Tract
Drugs That Act in the Lower GI Tract
  Inflammatory Bowel Disease

ORGANIZATION OF CLASS

The organization of these drugs is based on the organization of the gastrointestinal (GI) tract. There are drugs that are used in treating ulcers in the stomach and duodenum. There are also drugs that affect motility in the upper GI tract. Then, moving down to the large intestine, we can divide the agents into those that enhance motility and those that reduce motility. Finally, there are agents that specifically target diseases of the lower GI tract.

DRUGS THAT ACT IN THE UPPER GI TRACT

Orlistat is a lipase inhibitor being used to treat obesity.

Orlistat binds to pancreatic and gastric lipase and inactivates the enzyme. This reduces the absorption of dietary fat by about 30%. Adverse effects include flatulence, oily spotting, and fecal urgency.

Duodenal and gastric ulcers are often caused by the bacterium *Helicobacter pylori*. The treatment objective is eradication of *H. pylori* with a combination of antibiotics and H_2 blockers. Bismuth (PEPTO-BISMOL) appears to be bactericidal to *H. pylori*.

The "proton pump inhibitors" ("-prazoles") inhibit the H^+-K^+-ATPase enzyme of the parietal cell. This reduces acid secretion.
  OMEPRAZOLE
  ESOMEPRAZOLE
  dexlansoprazole (delayed-release formulation of the R-enantiomer of lansoprazole)
  lansoprazole
  pantoprazole
  rabeprazole

Proton pump inhibitors are used principally to promote healing of duodenal and gastric ulcers and in the treatment of GERD (gastric esophageal reflux disease).

> H_2 receptor antagonists prevent histamine-induced acid release. H_2 antagonists include:
> CIMETIDINE—watch out for drug interactions!
> RANITIDINE
> famotidine
> nizatidine

These drugs are easily recognizable by the "-tidine" ending. These drugs are used to promote healing of ulcers. Cimetidine binds to cytochrome P450. Therefore, adverse drug interactions with drugs transformed via the cytochrome P450 system are common with cimetidine.

> The aluminum salts and calcium carbonate antacids cause constipation. The magnesium salts cause diarrhea. Therefore, they are often mixed.

Antacids can decrease the absorption of other drugs because they alter the stomach and duodenal pH. They can also bind to drugs and block their absorption. This is particularly true for the aluminum salts. Antacids also have systemic effects. Magnesium salts can cause hypermagnesemia and aluminum salts can cause hypophosphatemia.

> SUCRALFATE forms a protective coating on the mucosa, particularly ulcerated areas.

Sucralfate is only minimally absorbed. Constipation is the main side effect.

> Metoclopramide and cisapride increase the rate of gastric emptying.

A diverse group of agents enhance coordination and increase transit of material in the GI tract. Cholinergic agonists (bethanechol) and acetylcholinesterase inhibitors, such as neostigmine, increase motility. Serotonin (5-HT) affects both secretion and motility. Metoclopramide is considered to act predominantly as an agonist at 5-HT_4 receptors. Cisapride has been removed from the market in the United States due to cardiac arrhythmias.

> MISOPROSTOL is a prostaglandin analogue that increases bicarbonate and mucin release and reduces acid secretion. It is used to treat nonsteroidal anti-inflammatory drug (NSAID)–induced ulceration.

Antiemetic drugs were covered in Chapter 37.

DRUGS THAT ACT IN THE LOWER GI TRACT

Diarrhea is most often caused by infection, toxins, or drugs. Bacterial or parasitic diarrhea should be treated with the appropriate agent for the infection. Drug-induced diarrhea should be treated by discontinuation of the drug, if possible. An example of targeted therapy for diarrhea is the use of octreotide (synthetic soma-tostatin) for the diarrhea associated with vasoactive intestinal peptide secreting tumors and metastatic carcinoid tumors (they secrete serotonin).

Opiates that are used to treat diarrhea include DIPHENOXYLATE and LOPERAMIDE. Eluxadoline is a μ receptor agonist and δ receptor antagonist that is approved for use in irritable bowel syndrome with diarrhea (IBS-D). These opiates should *not* be used for an infectious process. Antagonists of the 5-HT$_3$ receptor have been shown to also decrease transit in the GI tract. Alosetron and ondansetron have been used for IBS-D. There are also absorbent powders such as KAOPECTATE that are used in the treatment of diarrhea. Bismuth subsalicylate (PEPTO-BISMOL) may coat irritated mucosal surfaces.

Drugs used to treat constipation can be divided into two groups: the bulk-forming agents and the stimulants and cathartics. These drugs are generally taken orally. Some can be administered by insertion into the rectum.

Irritable bowel syndrome can be associated with either or both constipation (IBS-C) and diarrhea (IBS-D). Spasms of the smooth muscle can cause consider-able pain and are treated with antispasmodics, such as hyoscyamine or dicyclo-mine. These drugs have direct actions to cause muscle relaxation and are anticholinergic.

The bulk-forming agents used to treat constipation contain plant matter that absorbs water and softens the stool. These include:
 calcium polycarbophil
 methylcellulose
 psyllium

The stimulants used to treat constipation increase water and electrolytes in the feces and increase motility. These include:
 bisacodyl
 danthron
 phenolphthalein
 senna

You probably recognize these more by their trade names of METAMUCIL (psyllium), DULCOLAX (bisacodyl), and EX LAX (phenolphthalein). It helps to remember which are bulk-formers and which are stimulants.

There are a couple of others that you may be asked about. Salts of magne-sium and sodium (MILK OF MAGNESIA) draw water into the colon. Docusate (COLACE) improves penetration of water and fat into feces.

Lubiprostone, a prostaglandin E1 analogue, is approved for the treatment of chronic constipation and IBS-C. It activates chloride channels in the epithelium of the GI tract, stimulating intestinal fluid secretion.

Also approved for irritable bowel syndrome with constipation are the guanylate cyclase-C agonists (linaclotide and plecanatide), which bind to receptors on the epithelium of the intestine resulting in increased secretions into the lumen and accelerated transit and the NHE3 inhibitor tenapanor. NHE3 (in case you don't remember) is the sodium-hydrogen exchanger 3, which inhibits sodium reabsorption in the GI tract, resulting in acceleration of GI transit time. A 5-HT$_4$ agonist (tegaserod) was approved in 2002, removed from the market in 2007, and recently returned to the market for the treatment of IBS-C. As you, hopefully, remember from physiology, serotonin plays a major role in regulation of motility and secretions in the GI track. Activation of 5-HT$_4$ receptors stimulates secretion and increases transit.

INFLAMMATORY BOWEL DISEASE

Inflammatory bowel disease is generally divided into ulcerative colitis (confined to the colon) and Crohn disease (affects both small and large intestine). For both of these diseases consideration needs to be given to induction of remission and maintenance of remission. Sometimes the same drugs are used for both, but not always. These details are secondary to getting down the main drugs classes used for these conditions.

Inflammatory bowel disease can be treated by the following classes of drugs:
  Aminosalicylates
  Corticosteroids
  Immunosuppressants
  Tumor necrosis factor (TNF) inhibitors
  Integrin receptor antagonists
  Antibiotics

In the table above, see if you can list at least one drug for each category.

Primary therapy utilizes steroids and 5-aminosalicyclate (5-ASA), also called mesalamine, to control the inflammatory process. 5-ASA probably inhibits leukotriene production and has antiprostaglandin and antioxidant activity. Sulfasalazine, balsalazide and olsalazine (prodrugs for mesalamine), and mesalamine itself are used in mild to moderate ulcerative colitis and for maintenance of remission in ulcerative colitis.

Immunomodulating agents are also used in inflammatory bowel disease—including azathioprine, mercaptopurine, methotrexate, and cyclosporine (see Chapters 37 and 46). In addition, antibodies and antibody fragments that bind to tumor necrosis factor-α (TNF-α) block the inflammatory cascade and can be used in inflammatory bowel disease. Infliximab and adalimumab are monoclonal antibodies that bind to and inhibit TNF-α. Certolizumab pegol is an antibody fragment that is also used. These TNF-α inhibitors are generally reserved for disease refractory to more conventional therapy. Natalizumab and vedolizumab are monoclonal antibodies that are used in Crohn disease. They reduce intestinal inflammation by binding α_4 integrin, a molecule that mediates adhesion of leukocytes to endothelial receptors.

Nonnarcotic Analgesics and Anti-Inflammatory Drugs

45

- Organization of Class
- Nonsteroidal Anti-Inflammatory Drugs
- COX-2 Inhibitors
- Salicylates, Including Aspirin
- Acetaminophen
- Other Drugs for Arthritis
- Antigout Agents
- Drugs Used in the Treatment of Headaches

ORGANIZATION OF CLASS

Some textbooks put these drugs after the opiate analgesics and others group the antiarthritis drugs together. Basically, we will consider here some salient features of the nonnarcotic analgesics and some of the anti-inflammatory agents. I've also included the drugs used for gout and migraines. The largest group of drugs here is the nonsteroidal anti-inflammatory drugs (NSAIDs). This group includes aspirin and salicylates. However, the salicylates and aspirin have some important special features, so I have separated them to emphasize these features.

NONSTEROIDAL ANTI-INFLAMMATORY DRUGS

NSAIDs	
IBUPROFEN	meclofenamate
INDOMETHACIN	nabumetone
KETOROLAC	oxaprozin
NAPROXEN	phenylbutazone
diclofenac	piroxicam
etodolac	sulindac

(Continued)

NSAIDs (*Continued*)	
fenoprofen	suprofen
flurbiprofen	tolmetin
ketoprofen	
meloxicam	
mefenamic acid	

Compare this list with the one in your textbook or class handouts. There seems to be no rhyme or reason to the names.

> *All* the nonsteroidal anti-inflammatory drugs (NSAIDs) (including aspirin) are thought to exert their clinical effects by inhibiting prostaglandin synthesis.

The primary site of action is the cyclooxygenase (COX) enzyme, which catalyzes the conversion of arachidonic acid to prostaglandin and endoperoxide (Figure 45–1). Prostaglandins modulate components of inflammation. They also are involved in control of body temperature, pain transmission, platelet aggregation, and other effects. They are not stored by cells but are synthesized and released on demand. Their half-lives are only minutes long. Therefore, if you control the enzyme that makes prostaglandins, you control the prostaglandins themselves.

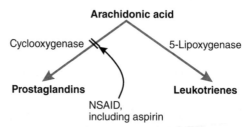

FIGURE 45–1 Remember that arachidonic acid is converted to both prostaglandins and leukotrienes. The nonsteroidal anti-inflammatory drugs (NSAIDs) inhibit the enzyme cyclooxygenase and, therefore, the formation of prostaglandins.

> *All* the NSAIDs (including aspirin) have analgesic, antipyretic, and anti-inflammatory effects. The older (nonspecific) NSAIDs also have antithrombotic effects.

The NSAIDs (including aspirin) are used in the treatment of moderate pain, fever, tendinitis, sunburn, rheumatoid arthritis, and osteoarthritis, just to name a few.

> The most common adverse effects of the NSAIDs (including aspirin) are gastrointestinal (GI) injury and renal injury.

Gastrointestinal (GI) injury consists of gastritis and ulcers. Misoprostol, a synthetic prostaglandin analogue, is used for the prevention of NSAID-induced ulcers. NSAIDs can cause oliguria, fluid retention, decreased sodium excretion, renal failure, and can prolong bleeding time.

The agents differ with respect to their central nervous system (CNS) side effects, duration of action, degree of platelet antagonism (bleeding), and GI toxicity.

> KETOROLAC is an NSAID that can be administered intramuscularly or intravenously. Ibuprofen and meloxicam are now also available for intravenous administration.

COX-2 INHIBITORS

Two isoforms of the COX enzyme have been identified. COX-1 is expressed constitutively in most tissues and is thought to protect the gastric mucosa. COX-2 is expressed constitutively in the brain and kidney and is induced at sites of inflammation. COX-1, but not COX-2, is present in platelets. The older NSAIDs block both COX isoforms. Theoretically, a specific COX-2 inhibitor should be anti-inflammatory without harming the GI tract or altering platelet function.

COX-2 inhibitors are all named with the ending "-coxib." They include celecoxib and rofecoxib.

SALICYLATES, INCLUDING ASPIRIN

> Aspirin causes irreversible inactivation of COX. It is the only NSAID to do this.

Aspirin and other salicylates are metabolized to salicylic acid, which is the active agent. Aspirin acetylates the COX enzyme, causing irreversible inactivation of the enzyme. Therefore, its effect lasts until the body makes more enzyme.

Aspirin brings down a fever, reduces minor pain and inflammation, and prevents blood clots. The antipyretic and analgesic actions are mediated by an action in the CNS. Aspirin is now also considered an essential element in the management of an acute myocardial infarction.

> Use of aspirin has been associated with Reye syndrome in children.

Reye syndrome is characterized by CNS damage, liver injury, and hypoglycemia. Its cause is unknown. The incidence of Reye syndrome has fallen dramatically with education of the public not to give aspirin to children.

> Overdose of aspirin is called salicylism. Symptoms include ringing in the ears (tinnitus), dizziness, headache, fever, and mental status changes.

Notice that overdose can cause the very symptoms that the patient set out to treat (headache, fever).

The pH changes after ingestion of large amounts of aspirin are complex, but important to understand.

1. Stimulation of the medullary respiratory center causes an increase in ventilation. This leads to *respiratory alkalosis* ($\uparrow$pH and $\downarrow$pCO$_2$).
2. There is uncoupling of oxidative phosphorylation. This leads to an increase in plasma CO$_2$, which further stimulates the respiratory center.

Aspirin has zero-order kinetics.

Remember zero-order kinetics? Aspirin and salicylic acid are metabolized by glucuronidation—an enzymatic reaction that can be saturated. Therefore, elimination can become zero-order (saturation kinetics). This is reflected in the plasma half-life, which increases with increasing doses. Also, aspirin is an example of a drug where the half-life does not match the duration of action. Why? Because, aspirin causes the irreversible inactivation of COX.

ACETAMINOPHEN

ACETAMINOPHEN has analgesic and antipyretic actions but does *not* have anti-inflammatory or antithrombotic activity.

Acetaminophen only weakly inhibits prostaglandin synthesis and has no effect on platelet aggregation.

ACETAMINOPHEN can cause *fatal* liver damage.

In overdose, the major concern is liver damage. This is apparently mediated by the binding of a toxic metabolite to the liver itself (Figure 45–2). Toxicity can be prevented by intravenous (IV) administration of sulfhydryl donors such as *N*-acetylcysteine, if treatment is initiated quickly.

OTHER DRUGS FOR ARTHRITIS

Disease-modifying antirheumatic drugs (DMARDs) are used early in the treatment of rheumatoid arthritis to prevent irreversible damage. Methotrexate (see Chapter 37), an antifolate, is usually the DMARD of choice. Hydroxychloroquine and sulfasalazine are safer alternatives that may be appropriate in mild cases. An NSAID or corticosteroid can be used as adjunct treatment. For moderate to severe disease, a biologic agent can be combined with a conventional DMARD.

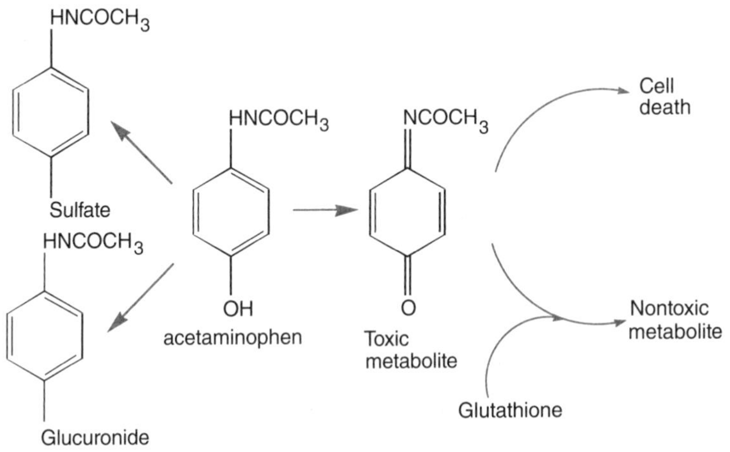

FIGURE 45-2 Acetaminophen can be metabolized in three directions (*arrows*). One direction gives a metabolite that is toxic to liver cells. However, glutathione can bind to the toxic metabolite and make it nontoxic. There are only limited quantities of glutathione available. Therefore, high doses of acetaminophen can be toxic.

Alternatively, a targeted synthetic DMARD, such as tofacitinib or baricitinib (Janus kinase inhibitors), can be used in patients with moderate to severe disease.

> Monoclonal antibodies used in the treatment of rheumatoid arthritis are antibodies to (largely) tumor necrosis factor-α (TNF-α) and interleukin 6 (IL-6).

Adalimumab, certolizumab, infliximab, and golimumab (obviously monoclonal antibodies) bind to tumor necrosis factor-α (TNF-α) and block the interaction of TNF-α with its receptors. Etanercept inhibits TNF-α by binding to and inactivating it. Remember that TNF-α is a naturally occurring cytokine that is involved in normal inflammatory and immune responses. Elevated levels of TNF-α are thought to play an important role in the inflammation and joint destruction in rheumatoid arthritis. These drugs are also used in inflammatory bowel disease (see Chapter 44). Tocilizumab and sarilumab are antibodies to the proinflammatory cytokine IL-6.

A variety of other antibodies and small molecules against inflammatory molecules are now available and more are likely to appear over the next several years. Tofacitinib, baricitinib, and upadacitinib are small molecule inhibitors of JAK enzymes. They are approved for moderate to severe rheumatoid arthritis. Rituximab is a monoclonal antibody against CD20, a surface antigen on B cells. Abatacept is a protein that interferes with T-cell activation.

ANTIGOUT AGENTS

Just a few facts here that you should be sure you know. Remember that gout is a buildup of uric acid in tissues. Inflammation is caused by migration of leukocytes to the joint in an attempt to clear away the uric acid crystals.

You need to distinguish between acute and chronic gout. For acute gout, colchicine, NSAIDs, or intra-articular glucocorticoids can be used. NSAIDs are the treatment of choice for acute flare-ups. IL-1 inhibitors, such as anakinra and canakinumab, have also been used to treat the pain and inflammation of acute gout.

> Colchicine can be used in acute attacks of gouty arthritis. It reduces inflammation.

Colchicine inhibits neutrophil activation. Hyperuricemia should be treated in patients with recurrent attacks and in those with chronic gout or evidence of tophi.

> ALLOPURINOL and febuxostat are urate-lowering agents that inhibit xanthine oxidase, thus reducing synthesis of uric acid.

Before starting treatment with urate-lowering agents, the patient should be free of all signs of inflammation. Pharmacologic treatment of hyperuricemia attempts to increase renal excretion of uric acid by decreasing tubular reabsorption or attempts to decrease synthesis of uric acid (Figure 45–3). Probenecid can be used to increase excretion of uric acid.

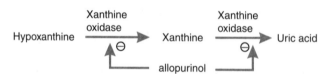

FIGURE 45–3 Uric acid is formed from hypoxanthine and xanthine by the enzyme xanthine oxidase. Allopurinol inhibits xanthine oxidase.

DRUGS USED IN THE TREATMENT OF HEADACHES

NSAIDs are the mainstay of the treatment of headaches, including migraines.

5-HT$_1$-Receptor Agonists ("-triptans")	
almotriptan	rizatriptan
eletriptan	sumatriptan
frovatriptan	ZOLMITRIPTAN
naratriptan	

The selective 5-HT$_1$-receptor agonists are highly effective for the treatment of acute migraine. A "-triptan" is the drug of choice for moderate to severe migraine pain in most patients. They act on intracranial blood vessels and peripheral sensory nerve endings, resulting in vasoconstriction and decreased release of inflamma-tory neuropeptides. Injectable and nasal forms of sumatriptan have faster onset of action than oral forms.

Calcitonin gene-related peptide (CGRP) is a potent vasodilator and neu-romodulator. Two small molecule CGRP receptor antagonists (rimegepant and ubrogepant) are approved for the acute treatment of migraine in adults. Another interesting drug is lasmiditan, a selective 5-HT$_{1F}$ receptor agonist, which binds to receptors on trigeminal neurons inhibiting pain pathways. Both the CGRP antag-onists and the 5-HT$_{1F}$ agonist can be used in patients with vascular disease.

The ergot alkaloids (dihydroergotamine and ergotamine) are most effective when taken early in an attack. If used frequently, a rebound headache can occur. These guys can have serious side effects.

A large number of compounds in a variety of drug classes have been used for prevention of migraine. None have achieved notable success. For continuous prophylaxis, β-blockers are most commonly used.

CHAPTER

46

Immunosuppressives

- Organization of Class
- Calcineurin Inhibitors
- Proliferation Signal Inhibitors
- Other Immunosupressants
- Biologics for Transplantation

ORGANIZATION OF CLASS

Immunopharmacology is the study of the use of drugs to modulate, usually depress, the immune response. These drugs are used in the treatment of autoimmune diseases (myasthenia gravis and rheumatoid arthritis) and in organ transplantation.

Glucocorticoids (see Chapter 38)
Calcineurin inhibitors
   CYCLOSPORINE
   tacrolimus
Proliferation signal inhibitors
   sirolimus
   everolimus
Other immunosuppressants
   mycophenolate mofetil
   thalidomide
   azathioprine
   cyclophosphamide
Biologics for transplantation
   belatacept
   daclizumab, basiliximab (anti-CD25)

CALCINEURIN INHIBITORS

CYCLOSPORINE inhibits antibody and cell-mediated immune responses and is the *drug of choice* for prevention of transplant rejection.

Cyclosporine (also ciclosporin) binds to cyclophilin (an intracellular protein of the immunophilin family), while tacrolimus binds to the immunophilin FK-binding protein and this complex inhibits calcineurin. So, link cyclosporine and tacrolimus in your head.

PROLIFERATION SIGNAL INHIBITORS

Sirolimus and its derivative everolimus bind to an immunophilin called protein called FK506-binding protein 12. This complex blocks the molecular target of rapamycin (mTOR), which leads to the inhibition of interleukin-driven T-cell proliferation.

OTHER IMMUNOSUPRESSANTS

Mycophenolate mofetil is administered as a prodrug that is activated to mycophenolic acid—the active compound. It is a highly selective inhibitor of a crucial enzyme in the de novo synthesis of guanosine. Proliferating lymphocytes are dependent on the de novo pathway for purine biosynthesis. Most other cell lines can maintain function with the salvage pathway. Therefore, mycophenolic acid is a very specific lymphocyte inhibitor.

Azathioprine (prodrug for mercaptopurine) is thought to be immunosuppressive by interfering with DNA synthesis. Azathioprine and cyclophosphamide you should remember from the anticancer drugs (see Chapter 37).

BIOLOGICS FOR TRANSPLANTATION

Basiliximab and daclizumab block the interleukin-2 (IL-2)–mediated activation of T lymphocytes by binding to CD25, which is the α chain of the interleukin-2 receptor. These antibodies were designed to selectively inhibit T-cell activation. Both are used to prevent rejection after organ transplantation.

Belatacept blocks T-cell stimulation and has been used in transplant medicine.

47 Drugs Used in Osteoporosis

Organization of Class

Bisphosphonates

Denosumab

Parathyroid Hormone

Selective Estrogen Receptor Modulators

Calcitonin

Sclerostin Inhibitor

ORGANIZATION OF CLASS

Some of the drugs for osteoporosis have been covered elsewhere, but many of these drugs do not fit into other categories, so this chapter was created to pull this information together in one place.

Osteoporosis is the term used for a set of diseases characterized by the loss of bone mass. It is the most common of the metabolic bone diseases and is an important cause of morbidity in the elderly.

> Pharmacologic therapy is targeted toward both prevention of bone loss and treatment of established osteoporosis (increasing bone mass and reducing fractures).

If you have not already done so, now is a good time to review the hormonal control of serum calcium and phosphorus concentrations. Which organs (kidney, parathyroid, intestine) produce which hormones that have what actions? Remember that bone is constantly forming and resorbing. The rates of the remodeling vary between people, between different bones, and at different ages. Diet and exercise play a major role in maintenance of bone mass. Intake of calcium and vitamin D are critical, and calcium supplements have been used for the treatment of osteoporosis. Calcium is not well absorbed from the gut and vitamin D improves absorption. Calcium supplementation has been shown to reduce bone loss in postmenopausal women, but not to increase bone density once lost. Calcium supplements are available in a variety of salts.

BISPHOSPHONATES

> ALENDRONATE
>
> ibandronate
>
> risedronate
>
> zoledronate

> The bisphosphonates inhibit osteoclastic activity and decrease bone turnover and resorption. They have been shown to reduce the incidence of fractures.

These agents inhibit farnesyl pyrophosphate synthase, an enzyme that appears to be critical for osteoclast survival. They have been shown to improve bone mass in established osteoporosis. They are not well absorbed from the gastrointestinal (GI) tract, and absorption is decreased even more by the presence of food. They bind to bone, thus having a lasting effect from a single dose. This is the basis of the once weekly or once yearly dosing now available. The half-life of alendronate in bone has been measured to be at least 10 years.

DENOSUMAB

Denosumab, a monoclonal antibody, is a RANK ligand inhibitor. RANK is "receptor activator of nuclear factor-κB." Denosumab prevents the interaction of the ligand with the receptor on cells of osteoclastic lineage. Remember that osteoclasts break down bone and activation of the RANK receptor stimulates osteoclasts. Thus, blocking this receptor will inhibit bone resorption.

PARATHYROID HORMONE

> Teriparatide (1-34) and abaloparatide (full-length), recombinant parathyroid hormone, are effective in reducing the incidence of new fractures in patients with osteoporosis.

Parathyroid hormone was reviewed in Chapter 40. Unlike other treatments for osteoporosis, teriparatide stimulates the formation of new bone and increases bone mass. It must be given by injection.

SELECTIVE ESTROGEN RECEPTOR MODULATORS

These compounds were introduced in Chapter 39. The selective estrogen receptor modulators have different degrees of estrogen agonist or antagonist activity in different tissues.

> Raloxifene and bazedoxifene have been approved for the prevention of postmeno-
> pausal osteoporosis.

Raloxifene is an estrogen agonist on bone and an antagonist in both the breast and uterus. Raloxifene has been shown to reduce the incidence of vertebral fractures without increasing the risk of breast or uterine cancer. It is not as effective as estrogen at increasing bone density. Like estrogen, the selective estrogen receptor modulators (SERMs) can increase the risk for thromboembolism.

CALCITONIN

Normally produced in the body, calcitonin regulates calcium levels by inhibiting osteoclastic activity (breakdown of bone). Calcitonin can be used in established osteoporosis, but studies have not shown a clear benefit to its use. It must be administered subcutaneously or by nasal spray. Calcitonin does have some analgesic action, which may be of benefit in patients with fractures.

SCLEROSTIN INHIBITOR

Romosozumab is a monoclonal antibody that binds to and inhibits sclerostin, a small protein expressed in osteocytes, thus increasing bone formation and decreasing resorption. It is given once a month by subcutaneous injection for up to a year.

Toxicology and Poisoning

Principles of Toxicology
General Principles in the Treatment of Poisoning
Specific Antidotes

PRINCIPLES OF TOXICOLOGY

> Toxicology is the study of the toxic or harmful effects of chemicals. It is also concerned with the symptoms and treatment of poisoning and the identification of the poison.

The variety of potential adverse effects and the diversity of chemicals in the environment make toxicology a very broad science. There are several fields of toxicology, including environmental (e.g., air and water pollution), economic (e.g., food additives, pesticides), legal (e.g., forensics, regulation of emissions, and additives), laboratory (e.g., analytical testing for chemicals), and biomedical (e.g., toxicities of drugs used to treat disease in humans and animals).

> The general principles of the toxic effects of chemicals are, for the most part, the same as the principles of the therapeutic effects of drugs.

GENERAL PRINCIPLES IN THE TREATMENT OF POISONING

Intentional and accidental poisonings are major medical problems. Every natural or synthetic chemical can cause injury if the dose is high enough.

> The single most important treatment of poisoned patients is supportive care.

This is so important. You must treat the patient and not the poison. Provide airway support and ventilation and support blood pressure if needed. Toxicology screens of blood or urine take time and rarely change your therapy. If you know the poison, great; if not, treat the patient.

> To reduce absorption in an alert, relatively asymptomatic patient, use activated charcoal.

To reduce the absorption of poisons from the gastrointestinal (GI) tract one can empty the stomach with gastric lavage, which needs to be carried out within 1 hours of ingestion, by administration of activated charcoal. Activated charcoal remains in the GI tract, absorbing poison throughout. Induction of emesis is no longer recommended.

To enhance elimination, a number of techniques can be used. Multiple doses of charcoal reduce the half-life and increase clearance. Increasing the pH of the urine enhances elimination of weak acids. Hemodialysis and hemoperfusion can be used to help remove specific agents from the blood.

SPECIFIC ANTIDOTES

For some overdoses and poisons, specific antidotes are available. These are prime examination material and are relatively easy to learn (some you already know).

Toxin	Antidote
acetaminophen	N-acetylcysteine
arsenic, mercury, gold	BAL (dimercaprol)
β-blocker	glucagon
benzodiazepines	flumazenil
carbon monoxide	oxygen, hyperbaric oxygen
coumarin	vitamin K
cyanide	nitrites
digoxin	digoxin-specific Fab fragments
ethylene glycol or methanol	fomepizole
heparin	protamine
iron	deferoxamine
isoniazid	pyridoxine
lead	dimercaprol, penicillamine, or succimer
narcotics	naloxone
nitrites	methylene blue
organophosphates	atropine, pralidoxime

Scan through this list and pick out the ones you already know. You should remember that flumazenil is the benzodiazepine receptor antagonist and that naloxone is the narcotic antagonist. You should know from biochemistry that oxygen and carbon monoxide compete for the same site on hemoglobin. You should remember from autonomics that pralidoxime rescues the acetylcholinesterase enzyme from the organophosphates. You should already know that vitamin K is the antidote for coumarin overdose, and protamine is the antidote for heparin overdose. So, there are really only a few new ones here.

Some of the antidotes directly bind or neutralize the poison. For instance, BAL (dimercaprol) chelates the metals, deferoxamine binds to iron, the monoclonal antibody to digoxin binds to the digoxin, and the nitrites neutralize cyanide. Dimercaprol, penicillamine, or succimer will all chelate lead. Both ethylene glycol and methanol are oxidized by alcohol dehydrogenase to toxic compounds. Fomepizole is a specific alcohol dehydrogenase inhibitor.

Index

A

abacavir, 170
abaloparatide, 237
abarelix, 187, 202
abatacept, 231
abciximab, 84
abemaciclib, 189
abiraterone, 187
acaclabrutinib, 189
acarbose, 211
ACE, 62, 69
acebutolol, 52
acetaminophen, 128, 230, 240
acetazolamide, 61, 124
acetophenazine, 113
acetylcholine, 28
acetylcholinesterase, 29, 37
aclidinium, 218
acrivastine, 215
ACTH, 193
actinomycin, 185
active transport, 10
acyclovir, 173
adalimumab, 226, 231
adefovir, 172
adenosine, 81
adrenal medulla, 29, 197
adrenaline, 29
afatinib, 189
aflibercept, 190
AIDS, 170
akathisia, 113
albiglutide, 209
albuteral, 46, 218
aldosterone, 62, 191
alectinib, 189
alendronate, 237
alfentanil, 126
alfuzosin, 52
alirocumab, 91
aliskiren, 64, 67
alkylating agents, 183
allergy, penicillin, 145
allopurinol, 232
almotriptan, 232

alogliptin, 209
alosetron, 224
alprazolam, 100
alteplase, 87
aluminum, 223
alvimopan, 126
amantadine, 118, 171
ambenonium, 37
ambrisentan, 220
amikacin, 150, 158
amiloride, 60
aminoglutethimide, 196
aminoglycosides, 140
aminosalicylic acid, 158
amiodarone, 80
amitriptyline, 107
amlodipine, 65, 72
amobarbital, 100
amoxicillin, 144
amphetamine, 47
amphotericin B, 163
ampicillin, 144
amylin, 211
anabolic, 28, 202
anakinra, 232
anastrozole, 187
androgens, 187
angiotensin, 62
angiotensin converting enzyme, 62
anidulafungin, 163
anistreplase, 87
antacids, 151
anthracyclines, 180
anticoagulant, 85
apalutamide, 187
apixaban, 85
aprepitant, 182
arachidonic acid, 228
ardeparin, 85
arecoline, 36
arformoterol, 218
argatroban, 85
aripiprazole, 113
arrhythmia, 77
arsenic, 240

artemether, 177
artemether-lumefantrine, 177
articaine, 134
asenapine, 113
asparaginase, 187
aspart, 208
aspirin, 72, 86, 128
astemizole, 216
asthma, 217
atazanavir, 170
atenolol, 52, 69
atezolizumab, 190
atomoxetine, 108
atorvastatin, 90
atracurium, 43
atropine, 39, 40, 82
autonomic nervous system, 27
avanafil, 203
avelumab, 190
avibactum, 143
axitinib, 190
azathioprine, 225, 235
azelastine, 215
azithromycin, 151
azlocillin, 144
azole antifungals, 163
azosemide, 58
aztreonam, 147

B

bacitracin, 147
baclofen, 119
bactericidal, 138
bacteriostatic, 138
baloxavir, 171
balsalazide, 225
bamlanivimab, 174
barbiturates, 100, 132
barbiturates, withdrawal, 102
baricitinib, 231
basiliximab, 235
bazedoxifene, 199, 238
beclomethasone, 219
belatacept, 235
bempedoic acid, 91

benazepril, 63
bendamustine, 183
bendroflumethiazide, 59
benralizumab, 220
benzathine pen G, 144
benznidazole, 176
benzocaine, 134
benzodiazepines, 100
benztropine, 41, 119
betamethasone, 193
betaxolol, 52
bethanechol, 36, 223
bevacizumab, 190
bicalutamide, 187, 198
bictegravir, 170
binimetinib, 189
bioavailability, 12
biperiden, 119
bisacodyl, 224
bismuth, 222
bisoprolol, 52, 69, 75
bivalirudin, 85
bleomycin, 183, 185
bortezomib, 190
bosentan, 220
bosutinib, 189
botulinum toxin, 43
bretylium, 80
brexpiprazole, 113
brivaracetam, 122
bromocriptine, 118
brompheniramine, 215
budesonide, 219
bumetanide, 58, 74
bupivacaine, 134
buprenorphine, 126
bupropion, 107
busprione, 100, 104
busulphan, 183
butoconazole, 163
butorphanol, 126

C
cabazitaxel, 185
cabozantinib, 189
calcineurin, 234
calcitonin, 238
calcium channel blockers, 64, 68, 81
calcium polycarbophil, 224
camptothecin, 185
canagliflozin, 211
canakinumab, 232
candesartan, 63, 73
capecitabine, 184
capreomycin, 158
captopril, 63, 73
carbachol, 36
carbamazepine, 111, 122
carbenicillin, 144
carbidopa, 117
carbon monoxide, 240
carboplatin, 183
cardiotoxicity, 182

carmustine, 183
carteolol, 52
carvedilol, 53, 69, 75
caspofungin, 163
catabolic, 28
catecholamine, 30
cefaclor, 146
cefamandole, 146
cefazolin, 145
cefepime, 146
cefotaxime, 146
cefoxitine, 146
cefpirome, 146
ceftazidime, 146
ceftriaxone, 146
celecoxib, 229
cell cycle, 181
cephalexin, 145
cephalosporins, 145
ceritinib, 189
certolizumab, 226, 231
cestodes, 166
cetirizine, 216
cetrorelix, 202
cetuximab, 188
cevimeline, 36
charcoal, 240
chlamydia, 151
chloral hydrate, 100
chlorambucil, 183
chloramphenicol, 153
chlordiazepoxide, 100, 103
chloroprocaine, 134
chloroquine, 177, 177
chlorothiazide, 59
chlorpheniramine, 215
chlorpromazine, 113
chlorprothixene, 113
cholera, 151
cholesterol, 90, 162
cholestyramine, 91
cholinesterase, 35, 97
cholinomimetic, 35
ciclesonide, 219
cidofovir, 173
cilastatin, 146
cilostazol, 88
cimetidine, 223
cinacalcet, 206
cinchonism, 178
ciprofloxacin, 156
cisapride, 223
cisatracurium, 43
cisplatin, 183
citalopram, 107
cladribine, 184
clarithromycin, 151
clavulanic acid, 143
clearance, 13
clemastine, 215
clindamycin, 150, 153
clofazimine, 161
clomiphene, 199

clonazepam, 100, 122
clonidine, 45, 49, 69
clopidogrel, 84
clorazepate, 100
clotrimazole, 163
cloxacillin, 144
clozapine, 113
cobicistat, 170
cobimetinib, 189
cocaine, 134
codeine, 126
colchicine, 232
colesevelam, 91
colestipol, 91
competitive antagonist, 7
COMT, 29, 118
cortisol, 193
cotrimoxazole, 155
coumarin, 240
craniosacral, 28
crizanlizumab, 89
crizotinib, 189
Crohn disease, 225
cromolyn, 220
cross-dependence, 100
cross-tolerance, 99
cyanide, 68, 240
cyanocobalamin, 89
cyclizine, 216
cyclooxygenase, 84, 232
cyclopentolate, 41
cyclophilin, 235
cyclophosphamide, 182, 234
cycloserine, 158
cyclosporine, 225, 234
cyproheptadine, 216
cyproterone, 198
cytarabine, 184

D
dabigatran, 85
dabrafenib, 189
dacarbaine, 183
daclatasvir, 172
daclizumab, 235
dactinomycin, 182, 185
dalbavancin, 147
dalfopristin, 152
dalteparin, 85
danaparoid, 85
danthron, 224
dantrolene, 43
dapagliflozin, 76, 211
dapsone, 161
daptomycin, 148
darifenacin, 41
darolutamide, 187
darunavir, 170
dasabuvir, 172
dasatinib, 189
daunomycin, 185
daunorubicin, 182, 185
deferoxamine, 240

degarelix, 187, 202
delafloxacin, 156
delavirdine, 170
demecarium, 37
demeclocycline, 150
denosumab, 237
dependence, 99
deprenyl, 118
desflurane, 130
desipramine, 107
desirudin, 85
desloratadine, 216
desvenlafaxine, 107
deutetrabenazine, 114
dexamethasone, 193
dexlansoprazole, 222
dexmedetomidine, 49
dexmethylphenidate, 47
dexrazoxane, 185
dezocine, 126
diabetes insipidus, 111, 211
diabetes mellitus, 207
diabetics, 51
diazepam, 64, 100
diclofenac, 227
dicloxacillin, 144
dicumarol, 85
dicyclomine, 41, 224
didanosine, 170
diethylcarbamazine, 166
diethylstilbestrol, 197, 199
digitalis, 75
digitoxin, 75
digoxin, 73, 81, 240
dihydroergotamine, 233
diltiazem, 65, 72, 81
dimenhydrinate, 215
dimercaprol, 240
diphenhydramine, 215
diphenoxylate, 128, 224
diphtheria, 152
dipyridamole, 84
disopyramide, 78
diuretics, 67, 74
dobutamine, 46
docetaxel, 185
dofetilide, 80
dolasetron, 182
dolutegravir, 170
donepezil, 37, 97
dopamine, 30, 48, 109
doravirine, 170
doripenem, 146
doxacurium, 43
doxazosin, 50, 68
doxercalciferol, 206
doxorubicin, 182, 189
doxycycline, 150, 177
dronabinol, 182
dronedarone, 80
drotrecogin alfa, 85
droxidopa, 47
dulaglutide, 209
duloxetine, 107

dupilumab, 220
durvalumab, 190
dutasteride, 198
dystonia, 114

E
echothiophate, 37
econazole, 163
edoxaban, 85
edrophonium, 37
efavirenz, 170
efficacy, 6
eflornithine, 176
elbasvir, 172
eletriptan, 232
elexacaftor, 221
eluxadoline, 224
elvitegravir, 170
empagliflozin, 76, 211
emtricitabine, 170
enalapril, 63, 73
encorafenib, 189
endometriosis, 194
enflurane, 129
enfuvirtide, 170
enoxaparin, 85
entacapone, 118
entecavir, 172
enzalutamide, 187
ephedrine, 47
epilepsy, 102, 123
epinephrine, 30, 47, 82
epirubicin, 185
eplerenone, 73
epoprostenol, 220
eprosartan, 63
eptifibatide, 84
ergosterol, 162
ergotamine, 233
erlotinib, 189
ertapenem, 146
erythromycin, 151
erythropoietin, 89, 182
escitalopram, 107
esketamine, 110
eslicarbazepine, 122
esmolol, 52, 69
esomeprazole, 222
estradiol, 197
estriol, 197
estrogen, 197
estrone, 197
eszopiclone, 100, 104
etanercept, 231
etesevimab, 174
ethacrynic acid, 58
ethambutol, 158
ethanol, 103
ethinyl estradiol, 197
ethionamide, 158
ethosuximide, 122
ethylene glycol, 240
etidocaine, 134
etodolac, 227

etomidate, 130
etoposide, 185
etravirine, 170
everolimus, 189, 235
evinacumab, 93
evolocumab, 91
exemestane, 187
exenatide, 209
extrapyramidal effects, 114
ezetimibe, 91

F
famciclovir, 173
famotidine, 223
febuxostat, 232
felbamate, 122
felodipine, 65
fenbendazole, 176
fenofibrate, 91
fenoldopam, 69
fenoprofen, 228
fentanyl, 126
fesoterodine, 41
fexofenadine, 216
filaria, 166
filgrastim, 181
finasteride, 198, 201
fingolimod, 119
flecainide, 78
fluconazole, 163
flucytosine, 163
fludarabine, 184
fludrocortisone, 193
flumazenil, 103, 240
fluorouracil, 184
fluoxetine, 107
fluoxymesterone, 194, 198
fluphenazine, 113
flurazepam, 100
flurbiprofen, 228
flutamide, 187, 198
fluticasone, 193, 219
fluvastatin, 90
folic acid, 89, 154
fomepizole, 240
fondaparinux, 85
formaldehyde, 157
formestane, 187
formoterol, 218
fosamprenavir, 170
fosfomycin, 148
fosinopril, 63, 73
fosphenytoin, 122
frovatriptan, 232
fulvestrant, 187
furosemide, 58, 74

G
GABA, 102
gabapentin, 122
galantamine, 37, 97
gallamine, 43
ganciclovir, 173
ganirelix, 202

gastric lavage, 244
gatifloxacin, 156
gefitinib, 189
gemcitabine, 184
gemfibrozil, 91
gemifloxacin, 156
gentamicin, 150
glargine, 208
glatirmer acetate, 119
glaucoma, 38
glecaprevir, 172
glimepiride, 209
glipizide, 209
glomerular filtration, 24
glucagon, 207, 240
glucocorticoid, 187, 194
glyburide, 209
glycopyrrolate, 41, 218
golimumab, 231
golodirsen, 119
goserelin, 187, 202
granisetron, 182
grazoprevir, 172
griseofulvin, 163
growth factors, 181, 215
guanabenz, 49, 69
guanfacine, 49, 69

H
haloperidol, 113
halothane, 129
headaches, 232
helminths, 166
heparin, 85, 240
heroin, 126
hirudin, 85
histamine, 215
histrelin, 202
HIV, 170
HMG CoA reductase, 90
hookworm, 166
hydralazine, 68
hydrochlorothiazide, 59
hydrocodone, 126
hydrocortisone, 193
hydromorphone, 126
hydroxychloroquine, 177, 230
hydroxyprogesterone, 198
hydroxyurea, 89, 187
hydroxyzine, 215
hyoscyamine, 224
hypercalcemia, 186

I
ibandronate, 237
ibrutinib, 189
ibuprofen, 227
ibutilide, 80
idarubicin, 185
idarucizumab, 87
idelalisib, 189
ifosfamide, 183
iloperidone, 113
iloprost, 220

imatinib, 189
imipenem, 146
imipramine, 107
indapamide, 59
indinavir, 170
indomethacin, 227
infliximab, 226, 231
influenza, 171
inhibitory concentration, 140
insulin, 208
insulin detemir, 208
insulin glulisine, 208
interferon, 119
interferon-alpha, 172
inverse agonist, 9
ipilimumab, 190
ipratropium, 41, 218
irbesartan, 63
irinotecan, 185
iron, 89, 185, 244
isavuconazole, 163
isocarboxazid, 107
isoflurane, 129
isoniazid, 139, 158, 240
isoproterenol, 45, 82
isosorbide dinitrate, 72
isosorbide mononitrate, 72
isosorbide-5-mononitrate, 72
isradipine, 65
istradefylline, 118
itraconazole, 163
ivabradine, 73, 76
ivacaftor, 221
ivermectin, 166
ixabepilone, 186

K
kanamycin, 159
ketamine, 130
ketoconazole, 163, 187, 196
ketoprofen, 228
ketorolac, 227, 233

L
labetalol, 53, 69
lacosamide, 122
lamivudine, 170, 172
lamotrigine, 111, 122
lanoteplase, 87
lansoprazole, 222
lapatinib, 189
lasmiditan, 233
lead, 240
ledipasvir, 172
lefamulin, 152
lemborexant, 105
lepirudin, 85
leprosy, 161
letrazole, 187
leucovorin, 184
leuprolide, 187, 202
levalbuterol, 218
levetiracetam, 122
levobunolol, 52

levobupivacaine, 134
levocetirizine, 216
levodopa, 117
levofloxacin, 156, 159
levomilnacipran, 107
levonorgestrel, 198
levorphanol, 126
levothyroxine, 205
lidocaine, 78, 134
linaclotide, 225
linagliptin, 209
lincomycin, 153
linezolid, 152
liothyronine, 205
liotrix, 205
lipoprotein, 89
liraglutide, 209
lisinopril, 63, 73
lispro, 208
lithium, 111
lixisenatide, 209
log kill, 181
lometrexol, 184
lomitapide, 93
lomustine, 183
loop diuretics, 58
loperamide, 128, 224
lopinavir, 170
loracarbef, 146
loratadine, 216
lorazepam, 100
losartan, 63, 73
lovastatin, 90
lubiprostone, 225
luliconazole, 163
lumacaftor, 221
lumefantrine, 177
lurasidone, 113
Lyme disease, 151

M
MAC, 131
macitentan, 220
major tranquilizers, 112
malaria, 176
malathion, 37
mannitol, 61
MAO inhibitors, 109
maraviroc, 170
mebendazole, 166
mechlorethamine, 183
meclizine, 215
meclofenamate, 227
medroxyprogesterone, 198
mefenamic acid, 228
mefloquine, 177
megestrol, 198
meloxicam, 228
melphalan, 183
memantine, 97
meperidine, 126
mepivacaine, 134
mepolizumab, 220
meprevir, 172

mercaptopurine, 184, 225
mercury, 244
meropenem, 146
mesalamine, 225
MESNA, 182
mesoridazine, 113
mestranol, 197
metaproterenol, 46
metformin, 210
methacholine, 36
methadone, 126
methanol, 240
methenamine, 157
methicillin, 144
methimazole, 205
methohexital, 100, 132
methotrexate, 154, 184, 230
methyclothiazide, 59
methylcellulose, 224
methyldopa, 69
methylene blue, 240
methylnaltrexone, 126
methylphenidate, 47
methylprednisolone, 193
methyltestosterone, 198
metoclopramide, 223
metocurine iodide, 43
metolazone, 59
metoprolol, 52, 69
metronidazole, 175
metyrapone, 196
mexiletine, 78
mezlocillin, 144
MIC, 140
micafungin, 163
miconazole, 163
midazolam, 132
midostaurin, 189
mifepristone, 198
miglitol, 211
migraines, 232
milnacipran, 107
miltefosine, 176
mineralocorticoid, 196, 194
minocycline, 150
minoxidil, 68
miosis, 33
mipomersen, 93
mirabegron, 46
mirtazapine, 107
misoprostol, 194, 223
mithramycin, 186
mitomycin, 185
mitotane, 187
mitoxantrone, 187
mivacurium, 43
moexipril, 63
mometasone, 219
monobactam, 147
montelukast, 219
morphine, 126
motion sickness, 216
moxifloxacin, 156, 159
mupirocin, 152

muscarine, 36
myasthenia gravis, 38
mycobacteria, 158
mycophenolate mofetil, 235
mycoplasma, 151
mydriasis, 33

N
N-acetylcysteine, 240
nabilone, 182
nabumetone, 227
nadolol, 52
nafarelin, 202
nafcillin, 144
nalbuphine, 126
nalidixic acid, 156
nalmefene, 126
naloxone, 126, 240
naltrexone, 126
naproxen, 227
naratriptan, 232
narcotic, withdrawal, 127
natalizumab, 226
nateglinide, 209
natpara, 206
nebivolol, 69, 76
necitumumab, 189
nefazodone, 107
nelfinavir, 170
nematodes, 166
neomycin, 150
neostigmine, 37, 223
nephrotoxicity, 58
neprilysin, 74
neratinib, 189
nesiritide, 61
netupitant, 182
neuraminidase, 171
neuroleptic malignant syndrome, 115
neuroleptics, 112
neurotoxicity, 150, 213
nevirapine, 170
niacin, 91
nicardipine, 65
nicotine, 37
nifedipine, 65
nifurtimox, 176
nilotinib, 189
nilutamide, 187, 198
nitazoxanide, 176
nitrates, 72, 203
nitric oxide, 203
nitrogen mustards, 180, 176
nitroglycerin, 72
nitroprusside, 68
nitrous oxide, 129
nivolumab, 190
nizatidine, 223
noncompetitive antagonist, 8
noradrenaline, 29
norepinephrine, 30, 47
norethindrone, 198
norfloxacin, 156
norgestrel, 198

nortriptyline, 107
NPH (insulin), 208
NSAID, 227
nusinersen, 120
nystatin, 163

O
ocrelizumab, 119
octreotide, 224
ofatumumab, 119
ofloxacin, 156
olanzapine, 113
olmesartan, 63
olodaterol, 218
olsalazine, 225
omadacycline, 150
omalizumab, 219
ombitasvir, 172
omeprazole, 222
onasemnogene abeparvovec, 120
ondansetron, 182, 224
opicapone, 118
optic neuritis, 160
oral contraceptives, 200
oritavancin, 147
orlistat, 222
oseltamivir, 171
osilodrostat, 196
osimertinib, 189
osteoporosis, 236
ototoxicity, 58, 147
oxacillin, 144
oxaliplatin, 183
oxaprozin, 227
oxazepam, 100
oxcarbazepine, 122
oxiconazole, 163
oxybutynin, 41
oxycodone, 126
oxymorphone, 126

P
PABA, 154
paclitaxel, 185
palbociclib, 189
paliperidone, 113
palivizumab, 173
palonosetron, 182
pancuronium, 43
panitumumab, 188
pantoprazole, 222
parasympathetic, 28
parathion, 37
paricalcitol, 206
paritaprevir, 172
parkinsonism, 113
paroxetine, 107
partial agonist, 5
partial pressure, 130
passive diffusion, 24
pazopanib, 190
pembrolizumab, 190
pemetrexed, 184
penbutolol, 52

penciclovir, 173
penicillamine, 240
penicillin G, 144
penicillin V, 144
penicillin-binding proteins, 142
penicillins, 144
pentamidine, 163, 176
pentazocine, 126
pentobarbital, 100
pentostatin, 184
pentoxifylline, 88
peramivir, 171
perampanel, 122
perindopril, 73
perphenazine, 113
pertussis, 152
pertuzumab, 189
phenelzine, 107
phenobarbital, 100, 122
phenolphthalein, 224
phenoxybenzamine, 50
phentolamine, 50
phenylbutazone, 227
phenylephrine, 45
phenylpropanolamine, 47
phenytoin, 78, 124
phenytoin, kinetics, 123
photosensitivity, 151
physostigmine, 37
pibrentasvir, 172
pilocarpine, 36
pindolol, 52
pinworm, 166
pioglitazone, 210
pipecuronium, 43
piperacillin, 144
pirenzepine, 41
piretanide, 58
piroxicam, 227
pitavastatin, 90
plasmodium, 176
plecanatide, 225
plerixafor, 182
plicamycin, 185
poisoning, 239
polyene antifungals, 163
ponatinib, 189
posaconazole, 163
potency, 6
pralatrexate, 184
pralidoxime, 39, 240
pramipexole, 118
pramlintide, 211
prasugrel, 84, 86
pravastatin, 90
prazosin, 50, 68
prednisolone, 193
prednisone, 193
prilocaine, 134
primaquine, 177, 177
primidone, 122
probenecid, 145
procainamide, 78
procaine, 134

procarbazine, 187
prochlorperazine, 113
progesterone, 198
prolactin, 113
promethazine, 215
propafenone, 78
propantheline, 41
propofol, 130
propoxyphene, 126
propranolol, 52, 69
propylthiouracil, 205
protamine, 86, 212, 240
protease inhibitors, 170
psyllium, 224
pyrazinamide, 160
pyridostigmine, 37
pyridoxine, 159, 240
pyrimethamine, 154, 177

Q
quazepam, 100
quetiapine, 113
quinapril, 63, 73
quinestrol, 197
quinidine, 78
quinine, 79, 177
quinolones, 156
quinupristin, 152

R
rabeprazole, 222
radioactive iodine, 205
raloxifene, 197, 199, 238
raltegravir, 170
raltitrexed, 184
ramelteon, 100, 105
ramipril, 63, 73
ramucirumab, 190
ranitidine, 223
rapamycin, , 235
rasagiline, 118
remdesivir, 174
remifentanil, 126
renin, 33
repaglinide, 209
resistance, bacterial, 138
reslizumab, 220
respiratory syncytial virus, 174
retapamulin, 152
reteplase, 87
retrovirus, 170
revefenacin, 218
reverse agonist, 9
reverse transcriptase inhibitors, 170
Reye syndrome, 229
ribavirin, 173
ribociclib, 189
ribosomes, 149
rifabutin, 159
rifampin, 158
rifapentine, 159
rilpivirine, 170
riluzole, 119
rimantadine, 171

rimegepant, 233
riociguat, 220
risedronate, 237
risperidone, 113
ritonavir, 170, 172
rituximab, 190, 235
rivaroxaban, 85
rivastigmine, 37, 97
rizatriptan, 232
Rocky Mountain Spotted Fever, 151
rocuronium, 43
rofecoxib, 229
roflumilast, 219
rolapitant, 182
romidepsin, 190
romosozumab, 238
ropinirole, 118
ropivacaine, 134
rosiglitazone, 210
rosuvastatin, 90
rotigotine, 118
roundworms, 166
ruxolitinib, 189

S
sacubitril, 73
safinamide, 118
salicylism, 229
salmeterol, 218
saquinavir, 170
sargramostim, 182
sarilumab, 231
sarin, 37
saxagliptin, 209
schistosomiasis, 166
scopolamine, 41
secobarbital, 100
selegiline, 118
selexipag, 220
semaglutide, 209
senna, 224
sertraline, 107
sevoflurane, 130
sibutramine, 110
sickle cell disease, 89
sildenafil, 203, 220
silodosin, 50
simvastatin, 90
siponimod, 119
sirolimus, 189, 235
sitagliptin, 209
sofosbuvir, 172
solifenacin, 41
soman, 37
sorafenib, 190
sotalol, 80
spectrum, 138
spirochetes, 151
spironolactone, 60, 67, 73
SSRIs, 107
stavudine, 170
stibogluconate, 176
streptokinase, 87
streptomycin, 150, 159

succimer, 240
succinylcholine, 43
sucralfate, 223
sufentanil, 126
sugammadex, 43
sulbactam, 143
sulfacetamide, 155
sulfadiazine, 155
sulfamethoxazole, 155
sulfapyridine, 155
sulfasalazine, 155, 225, 230
sulfisoxazole, 155
sulfonamides, 140
sulindac, 227
sumatriptan, 232
sunitinib, 190
superinfection, 139
suprofen, 228
suramin, 176
suvorexant, 105
sympathetic, 28

T
t-PA, 87
tacrine, 97
tacrolimus, 235
tadalafil, 203, 220
tafenoquine, 177
tamoxifen, 187, 197, 203
tamsulosin, 50
tapentadol, 126
tapeworms, 166
tardive dyskinesia, 113
tasimelteon, 105
tavaborole, 165
tazobactam, 147
tedizolid, 152
tegaserod, 225
teicoplanin, 147
telavancin, 147
telbivudine, 172
telithromycin, 152
telmisartan, 63
temazepam, 100
temozolomide, 183
temsirolimus, 189
tenapanor, 225
tenecteplase, 87
tenofovir, 170, 172
terazosin, 50, 66
terbinafine, 163
terbutaline, 46
terconazole, 163
teriflunomide, 119
teriparatide, 206, 237
testolactone, 198
testosterone, 198, 201
tetrabenazine, 114
tetracaine, 134
tetracycline, 150
tezacaftor, 221
theophylline, 218
therapeutic index, 7

therapeutic window, 7
thiazide diuretics, 59
thioguanine, 184
thiopental, 100, 130
thioridazine, 113
thiotepa, 183
thiothixene, 113
thoracolumbar, 28
thyroglobulin, 204
tiagabine, 122
ticagrelor, 84, 86
ticarcillin, 144
ticlopidine, 84
tigecycline, 151
timolol, 52, 69
tinidazole, 176
tinzaparin, 85
tiotropium, 42, 218
tipranavir, 170
tirofiban, 84
tizanidine, 49, 119
tobramycin, 150
tocainide, 78
tocilizumab, 231
tofacitinib, 231
tolazoline, 50
tolcapone, 118
tolerance, 99
tolmetin, 228
tolnaftate, 163
tolterodine, 41
topiramate, 122
topotecan, 185
toremifene, 187, 197
torsemide, 58, 74
toxicology, 239
tramadol, 126
trametinib, 189
trandolapril, 63, 73
transposon, 139
tranylcypromine, 107
trastuzumab, 189
trazodone, 107
trematode, 166
treprostinil, 220
tretinoin, 194
triamcinolone, 193, 219
triamterene, 60
triazolam, 100
trifluoperazine, 113
trihexyphenidyl, 41, 119
trimazosin, 50
trimethoprim, 140, 155
triptorelin, 187, 202
tropicamide, 41
trospium, 41
tuberculosis, 158
tubocurarine, 43
tubular reabsorption, 24
tubular secretion, 24
tubulin, 167
tucatinib, 189

U
ubrogepant, 233
ulcerative colitis, 225
umeclidinium, 218
upadacitinib, 231
urokinase, 87

V
valacyclovir, 173
valbenazine, 114
valganciclovir, 173
valproate, 122
valsartan, 63, 73
vancomycin, 147
vandetanib, 189
vardenafil, 203
vecuronium, 43
vedolizumab, 226
velpatasvir, 172
vemurafenib, 189
venetoclax, 190
venlafaxine, 107
verapamil, 65, 72, 81
vibegron, 46
vidarabine, 173
vilazodone, 107
viltolarsen, 119
vinblastine, 185
vincristine, 182, 185
vinorelbine, 185
vitamin K, 86, 240
VMAT2, 114
voglibose, 211
vorapaxar, 85
voriconazole, 163
vorinostat, 190
vortioxetine, 107
voxelotor, 89

W
warfarin, 85
whipworm, 167
withdrawal, 100

Y
yohimbine, 51

Z
zafirlukast, 219
zaleplon, 100, 104
zanamivir, 171
zero order, 123
zidovudine, 170
zileuton, 219
ziprasidone, 113
zoledronate, 237
zolmitriptan, 232
zolpidem, 100, 104
zonisamide, 122